<u>Why Quantum Physicists Don't Get Fat</u>

Put the Science of Quantum Physics to Work for You; Inject Your Diet with Rocket Fuel!

By Greg Kuhn

Table of Contents

Part Two: How to Use Quantum Physics for Long-Term
Weight Loss

Chapter One -Forward

By Doreen Banaszack
Author of <u>Excuse Me, Your Life is Now</u>
Deliberate Creation Coach
www.doreenbanaszack.com

As a teacher of deliberate creation, author, and coach I am always excited to hear new voices in the field of human growth and potential. Especially when that voice is intelligent, articulate, and brings fresh and insightful perspectives! Greg Kuhn's voice is just that voice destined to help thousands of people to not only lose weight, but to expand and grow in any area of their lives. This is why I can guarantee that you are going to love and benefit greatly from <u>Why Quantum Physicists Don't Get Fat</u>.

When I first met Greg he explained that he is a futurist who helps people transform difficult challenges by re-framing their paradigms through the science of quantum physics. I was lucky enough to get an early copy of this manuscript and the more I read the more I realized he'd sold himself way short. After actually finishing the book I knew that Greg was going to end up becoming one of the growing body of teachers helping to usher in a new golden age of human growth. That's why I have been eagerly encouraging Greg to get this book into your hands ever since!

Greg's teachings about how to create a better, more desirable body are unique and truly transformational. Greg teaches that, with simple changes to the way you see the world, based on the super-accurate (and super-strange) science of quantum physics, your ideal body is a lot easier to achieve than you've probably thought previously.

Greg's writing is profound, yet it is also accessible, fun, and easy to read. I have read a lot about quantum physics and I can honestly say that Greg's explanation was the easiest to comprehend that I have come across. What is more important to me than Greg's ability to relate this information, however, is his loving spirit and genuine desire to help you. Trust me, you won't be able to not feel this desire coming off every page and that's exactly what makes this book so powerful.

The great news is that Greg is far from done! He has told me that this is the first in a series of self-help books which use quantum physics to solve many difficult challenges you may encounter. Please join me in encouraging Greg not to hold back! After reading, <u>Why Quantum Physicists Don't Get Fat</u> I trust you'll also join me in calling Greg an essential teacher as he helps you finally find your elusive ideal body.

Chapter Two – Preface

Since the mid 1990s, I have been working and writing with my father, Clifford C. Kuhn, M.D., a.k.a. the Laugh Doctor. Dr. Kuhn is a physician, medical school professor, comedian, and corporate trainer who helps people enhance their performance and health by creating a lighter attitude about themselves. In addition to being Dr. Kuhn's right-hand-man and most trusted collaborator, I'm a lifelong science geek who spent 15 years researching quantum physics and applying its principles to shed unwanted pounds and achieve my ideal body. In this book, I'll show you how to do the same for yourself.

But first, a little about where I am now. I am 44 years old and, in addition to my writing, I have a busy, full-time profession, I am a husband, a step-father, and I am the primary caregiver for my three sons. After applying the science of quantum physics to my own diet and exercise routine, I can now wear the same pants size I wore in high school and, believe it or not, take my shirt off at the pool without feeling embarrassment. I often get pegged as being 10 years younger than I am because of my lack of body fat (although the increasing salt-and-pepper color of my hair means that happens less often now). And while that's a description of how I look, it's how I *feel* that's really most important to me.

So how *do* I feel? And how might *you*, too, feel when you use the principles of quantum physics to reach your ideal weight? If you're like me, you'll feel:

Strong: Able to climb hills and stairs without losing your breath

Desirable: People give you second looks

Confident: You have a physical asset – your body – that far outshines any expensive wardrobe

Penny-wise: No longer do you have to buy new clothes just to get a better fit for your expanding body

Excited: About buying new clothes to fit your *shrinking* body (don't worry, you can get them on sale)

Attractive: And often mistaken for someone 10 years younger than you are

<u>Healthy</u>: You look in the mirror and your belly is gone

<u>Proud</u>: Friends and family see you and exclaim, "Wow! How much have you lost?!"

But I didn't always feel like this. When I left college, I started gaining weight little by little. You know how it works. My weight gain was gradual and insidious. By the time I was 28 years old, I had a growing spare tire of flab around my gut and I was trying every trick and fad on the market to shrink it – to no avail! In fact, had it not been for an innocent comment from my mother-in-law, I have no doubt I was headed for obesity.

On August 8th, 1996, I stepped onto some bathroom scales holding my four-month-old son so I could weigh him. My mother-in-law tallied our combined weight, and then I handed my son to my wife. My mother-in-law next recorded my weight alone so she could subtract it from the first total to get my son's. As she did so, she said, "You weigh 194 pounds, Greg. You've *really* put on some weight, haven't you?" (For reference, I am 5'11")

Her comment, while meaning no harm, really hurt; I was overly sensitive about my weight, because she was right. Just three years earlier, I had weighed in the vicinity of 160 pounds. And I had spent the last three years actively and purposefully trying to keep the expanding fat off me. Drinking water, starving myself, skipping meals, eating no fat, eating only certain types of food, taking vitamins, taking diet pills, punishing myself with exercise – you name it, I'd done it.

And, yet, here I was: three years later and 30-some pounds heavier with a growing (and, now we know, dangerous) spare-tire of flab around my midsection. My mother-in-law was right, and it seemed there was nothing I could do to stop it! I was fat and getting fatter, despite my best efforts. Compounding the problem, my best efforts were not only failing to keep fat off of me, they were making me miserable too. I often felt like a total failure and completely defeated.

I could have resigned myself to the inevitable, telling myself that this is just what happens to people as they age. But, for some reason, I did not give up that day and seek comfort in a doughnut or two (as was my habit at the time). For some reason, I was, instead, filled with resolve to change my life.

I resolved on that day to find a new way to live so that I would never have to diet again! I resolved to find a lifestyle that allowed me to feel good about myself and my body, so that I never had to look in the mirror and feel shame or disgust again. And since 1996 I have been creating, refining, and fine-tuning that very lifestyle.

My resolve dovetailed perfectly with the research and writing I was already doing for my father, exploring all the ways that humor could help improve one's physical health and mental outlook. Shortly after I began specific research on weight loss, I got a tip to check out the science of quantum physics and immediately saw its potential to change my life on a personal basis. I began to write about using quantum physics (and my father's prescription for humor) to lose weight. But more importantly, I began to *personally practice* using quantum physics to lose weight.

Since then, I have not only been able to create this plan (through exhaustive research, extensive trials, and even many errors), but my Dad and I have also been able to teach many others to use it as well. The science this plan is based upon is as infallible as any mankind has created, and you will soon find that using the principles of quantum physics will turn any diet or exercise program into that magical weight-loss formula you were originally promised.

As my Father and I both solved our weight problems using the approach described in this book, we both developed rock-solid confidence in the plan. My research was sound; this plan will always deliver weight loss because it is based upon the most infinitely reliable science yet created, quantum physics. If this plan failed you, I would expect nothing less than the law of gravity to fail you next!

I'm excited that you are picking this up today. I've already made all the mistakes and corrected them for you. All you have to do is start following the plan.

Chapter Three – Introduction

"The second assault on the same problem should come from a totally different direction."

Tom Hirshfield
Physicist

What I'm going to teach you about getting a better body is based on the very precise science of quantum physics. And to properly teach you these revolutionary concepts, I'm asking for both your patience and your willingness to learn. You should know in advance that some of the things I will teach you might make you uncomfortable because they may completely violate everything you "know" about how you, and the very world you live in, actually function.

Your reward for your patience and willingness to learn something new will be a complete understanding of not only *what* to do to finally attain your ideal body, but also *why* you are doing it. Knowing why you are doing it, in my experience, will remove most of the self-defeating fear and doubt that will undoubtedly creep up from time to time. As Peter Medawar, Nobel Prize-winning biologist said, "The human mind treats a new idea the way a body treats a strange protein – it rejects it."

Achieving your ideal body depends on accurately understanding how you function, how this universe functions, and how you interact with this universe. I also believe your investment in knowing both "why" and "how" this plan works will provide you the best opportunity to live it completely. And if you completely embrace this simple and easy plan, there is no way you can fail to achieve your goals!

I willingly confess that I am both a science and a history geek. In fact, my personal interest and life-long research in these fields is a big reason I've been able to joyfully create this blueprint for your ideal body. But I've tried my best to present only the science and history I believe you *need* to know in order to get the best results from your diet and exercise plan.

Another thing you should know is that my weight loss plan is very simple and easy to follow. Don't let the plan's simplicity and ease fool you into taking it lightly, though; this plan works better than some of the most complicated diet and exercise plans available.

So if you're sick and tired of your body in its current condition, you've found the right source. Whether you're motivated by a desire to finally feel healthy and lean or by a desire to look like you used to, you will find answers here. And they will work for you.

It is my personal wish that this book blesses you and your body beyond measure. And, of course, that it helps you lose as much weight as you ever dreamed. And I believe it will do both things. Thank you for sharing your energy and intention with me; I am honored to be a part of the new life you are creating for yourself – starting today.

Part One of Why Quantum Physicists Don't Get Fat: Why Quantum Physics Matters in Your Weight Loss Success

"Every great advance in science has issued from a new audacity of imagination."

John Dewey
Scientist

Whether or not you consciously think about it every day, there is nothing that impacts your life more than science. Even if you didn't like studying science in school and don't care if you never learn anything about it again, the life you lead is almost entirely the creation of science.

I'm not referencing all the wonderful inventions and improvements which have made a positive impact on your daily life when I make that claim; I'm talking about an influence much deeper than gadgets and technology that make your life more comfortable, productive, and enjoyable. Science influences your life beyond the inclusion of flat screen televisions, cell phones, and iPads. Science is the reason you believe the things you do, the reason you see things the way you do, and the reason you do the things you do. Science creates your paradigms.

Historian Thomas Kuhn coined the term "paradigm" in his 1962 book, The Structure of Scientific Revolutions. He argued that scientists must always be aware of paradigm shifts which open up new ways of understanding things that they may not have previously considered valid. The terms "paradigm" and "paradigm shift" are now in our everyday lexicon and are applied now to anyone, scientist or not.

Put in layman's terms, a paradigm is your framework, or lens, through which you understand the world. It might help you to think of your paradigms as the web browsing software you use. Everyday you visit a vast array of websites, for personal, business, and entertainment purposes, and they are all distinct and unique. But your web browser (whether Internet Explorer, Google Chrome, or any other you might use) is always the constant framework for all the websites you visit, providing the structure for their use and display; you might not even have realized this, but a website often looks and functions completely differently in different web browsers. The web browser you use presents the web sites to you in a certain format and provides you with unique web surfing options (which are different from other web browsers) while browsing the Internet.

You probably don't ever think about which web browser you use because you are accustomed to it and it is familiar to you. You wouldn't really ever have any reason to think about which web browser you use either because the one you use works just fine for you – you get to the web sites you want to visit and you're able to do everything you want to on the Internet. Why would you think about it?

But what if your web browser didn't work for you anymore? What if you weren't able to visit the web sites you wanted to go to, what if you couldn't purchase the items on the Internet you wanted, or what if you could no longer do the things you wanted to on the Internet, like being unable to connect with friends via email or social networking sites?

Your first thought might be to tinker and experiment with the particular websites you've been using. But what if, no matter how many different websites you tried, you still couldn't do the things you wanted to on the Internet? You might consult a tech-savvy friend and that friend might tell you something like, "The web browser you're using is too limited; you should install Google Chrome (for example) and start using it to surf the web."

Your learned friend, it turns out, would probably be correct. If you followed her advice, you would have to go through a slightly awkward adjustment period where you became accustomed to the new ways that Google Chrome worked and got familiar with the new format. But, once you were familiar with the new web browser, you would realize that the slight inconvenience of learning the new ways of operating it was worth it because you could now do all the things you want to on the Internet.

That is exactly how paradigms work. If you replace "web browser" with "paradigm" in the previous example, and replace "do the things you want to on the Internet" with "lose weight", you will have a good illustration of how a new paradigm will work for you. In the previous example, the "websites you're visiting" can be replaced with "your weight loss plans and programs." Just like using a new web browser would suddenly allow you to do exactly what you want to on the Internet, with new paradigms you'll find that your weight loss efforts suddenly become super effective.

If you're like me, you'll even find that with new paradigms, your weight loss efforts become more effective than you were originally promised!

Because, if you're reading this book, your "web browser" (of course, I am referring to your "paradigms") is not allowing you to "use the Internet" (and, of course, I really mean "lose your unwanted weight") the way you want. It's time to consult your "tech savvy friend" (in this case, I am really referring to Why Quantum Physicists Don't Get Fat) and get a new "web browser" (once again, I really mean "paradigms") so that you can "do what you want on the Internet" (again, "lose your unwanted weight").

Your old paradigms have failed you in your continued quest to lose your unwanted weight (and you'll soon learn why…hint – don't blame yourself because it's not *your* fault) and it's time for new ones (which you are about to learn and are infinitely more effective)!

And, since our paradigms are created from science, learning about quantum physics will be the single greatest investment you'll ever make for losing weight. Quantum physics, you'll soon learn, is an amazing and supremely accurate science which shows us that we should completely rethink everything we thought we knew about how the universe operates. And the changes which you'll make from it are easy, fun, and incredibly effective for weight loss!

I will not force you to learn any boring or unnecessary science in this book. But I will give you an overview of quantum physics and the new paradigms it creates for you – so you can use the new paradigms to achieve a body of your dreams. If you are adamant about not reading about this science right now, you can skip Part One of <u>Why Quantum Physicists Don't Get Fat</u> and go directly to Part Two. Part Two is devoted to putting these new paradigms to use.

But if you do choose to skip Part One for now, I urge you to return to Part One when you finish. Part One of this book is entertaining and enlightening, but more importantly, Part One will arm you with vital information about why you're doing what you're doing with your new paradigms. And, because everyone experiences some slight discomfort when making changes (especially changes to the way you've been doing things your entire life), Part One will be invaluable as you experience the normal doubts and ups-and-downs which accompany any change.

Chapter Four - The "What If...?" Game

"A scientific truth does not triumph by convincing its opponents and making them see the light, but rather because its opponents eventually die and a new generation grows up that is familiar with it."

Maxwell Plank
Physicist
Nobel Prize Winner

To illustrate how our understanding of science has changed over the centuries, let's play a little game I call "What if...?". To play the game, imagine returning to an earlier time in history but with attributes you currently possess. For example, what if you could go back to high school but have your current level of maturity and wisdom? Imagine how you'd rule your high school under those circumstances. (I'd be like a superhuman compared to my teenage peers, and I'd finally get to be the homecoming king!)

Or what if you could live at the beginning of the scientific revolution but possess our modern understanding of science and the way our universe operates? You would truly be an intellectual giant, capable of amassing vast personal wealth and success, wouldn't you? And not only that, you'd probably be able to help thousands of other people, too.

Before the scientific revolution, everyone believed that:

- All of existence was a moment-to-moment, renewable miracle, and God's divine power was the one and only cause or explanation for any of it.
- There were only four elements on Earth, and all things here were made of them: air, fire, earth, and water.
- Fire and air, being lightweight, naturally traveled upward, above the Earth, and combined to form a fifth element called aether.
- Everything not on the Earth (stars, planets, moon, etc.) was made of aether.

- The Earth was the center of the universe; the Sun and the planets revolved around the Earth in epicycles.
- The one and only cause of all planetary motion was God's divine power.

Before the scientific revolution was fully integrated into the world, even the most learned, educated, and successful people considered these "facts" to be absolute truths, and everything in their world was predicated upon beliefs culled from such facts. Strange practices and beliefs were commonplace:

- People wrapped urine-soaked hose around their neck to fight off colds.
- People thought that the planets moved around in the "universal aether" because they were being pushed by angels.
- Surgeons carved holes in skulls to cure migraines, seizures, and mental illness.
- Beaver testicles were ground up and mixed with alcohol as a female contraceptive.
- Mercury, a deadly poison, was applied externally to cure wounds and consumed

internally to cure a wide variety of ailments such as constipation.

- People believed that bad smells and malodorous vapors caused illness.
- Women rubbed puppy urine on their faces as a beauty treatment (and even brushed their teeth with it).
- Farmers believed that having sexual intercourse under an evergreen tree produced abundant and fertile harvests.

In our "What if...?" fantasy, you alone would see these beliefs for what they were: superstition that was nonsensical at best and harmful at worst, based upon erroneous understandings of the physical world.

Today, even though many of us do still believe in God and God's power, we also acknowledge proven scientific facts that govern our natural world. Forces and materials such as gravity, matter, elements, chemical reactions, and other verifiable phenomena are known, undisputed, and accepted as active agents in our universe.

Now here's the really interesting part – and the purpose for our playing this game: We are currently in the middle stages of a <u>second</u> scientific revolution. But don't worry if you didn't know that. Just as there was no announcement during the first scientific revolution of the 17th century, there has been no official announcement today. Nobody has broadcast:

"Attention everyone! Attention everyone! We are in the middle of the second scientific revolution! Get ready, because your entire life will be changing!"

Even unannounced, however, the scope of the second scientific revolution almost makes the first one look like the work of primary students. It's that much more important and that much more significant!

And, through this book, you will actually be able to live out the "What if…?" fantasy in regards to achieving the phenomenal and desirable body of your dreams. The ideas you learn here may sound strange to you – stranger, perhaps, than hearing that the Earth revolved around the sun would have sounded to a person living during the early 17th century. But these new ideas are *true* and they are *real,* even though they're radically different from what you currently know.

"For those not shocked when they first come across quantum theory cannot possibly have understood it."

Niels Bohr
Physicist
Nobel Prize Winner

Now you get to play the "What if…?" game *in your real life.* You will be one of a growing number of people who are using the findings of the second scientific revolution to change their life <u>now</u> (instead of 100 years from now). The things you're about to learn will become the conventional wisdom of the future. Using these "facts of the future" before they become commonplace will allow you (with a little practice) to easily secure your ideal body, great health, and a sense of personal triumph.

Chapter Five - The First Scientific Revolution: Classical Physics and How it Shaped Our Thinking

"I have noticed that even people who claim everything is predetermined and that we can do nothing to change it, look before they cross the road."

Stephen Hawking
Physicist
Nobel Prize Winner

To illustrate how the faulty science of the first scientific revolution has hindered your weight loss efforts, let's begin with a short quiz:

1. When you don't like how much you weigh, do you try to identify the outside factors – such as the foods you're eating – that are causing the problem?

2. Have you ever referred to yourself as if you're a machine, using phrases like "I need to get myself operating better"?

3. Do you believe that certain food compounds, like fats, carbohydrates, or sugar, are bad for your body and will always have the same negative effects upon it?

4. Have you ever listened to the voice inside your head and thought of that voice as "you"?

5. When you want to lose weight, is your first instinct to take action (like eating less or eating different foods) to initiate that change?

6. Do you believe that following certain rules about the foods you eat or your exercise program will have predictable and reliable weight loss results?

7. Do you think it's unfair that you weigh too much because, after all, you want to lose weight so badly and you work hard at following your weight loss plan?

8. Have you ever allowed other people's expectations or reactions to influence

how you feel about yourself or your weight?

9. Do you count calories or try to limit the amount of fat you eat in an effort to lose weight?

If you answered "yes" to any of these questions, you can thank none other than good old Sir Isaac Newton. Yep, Newton, the father of the first scientific revolution, helped discover all the scientific facts upon which these beliefs are based. And they're all good examples of how we've interpreted and integrated his discoveries into our everyday lives.

There is no dispute that the first scientific revolution changed the entire world. For almost three hundred years, it seemed that scientists during the first scientific revolution had figured out, once and for all, how the *entire universe* operated. In fact, by the late 1800's, physicist Lord Kelvin (famous for his discovery of absolute zero) was advising his best students to pursue a field of study other than physics because "…all the interesting work has been done here." And, of equal importance, the first scientific revolution allowed people to separate science from theology, giving people permission to learn everything they could about the natural world.

Newton and the first scientific revolution determined the following four seminal truths about the universe, and we've based almost all of our understanding of how the world works upon them.

- Each "thing" (including the universe itself) is made of smaller parts with predictable functions. The smaller parts play roles in making the larger thing work. That is their "job."

- For every action, there is an equal and opposite reaction. Every movement has a cause. Every action is determined by something else exerting itself upon the thing that acted.

- The observer and the observed are two separate things. A scientist, a teacher, a manager, an administrator, etc., are all distinct and separate observers of what they are observing or experimenting with.

- Things occur in a logical, linear fashion. When a certain outcome occurs, you can always find the cause by tracing the multiplied effects backwards. Action is like a row of dominoes falling after the first one gets pushed.

Those four rules were enough, by themselves, to change everything in the world. How is that possible? Because after scientists proved these rules and shared them with the world at large, the rest of the world systematically studied how they applied to, and altered, every field outside the world of science. The rest of the world used these new rules to create new paradigms – ways of viewing the world – and those paradigms are what caused you to answer "yes" to one or more of the questions in our short quiz.

Before we examine how those beliefs manifest in our modern lives – and in our attempts to lose weight – let's talk about paradigms for a moment. A paradigm is the lens through which you see and understand the world. It is your filter and your basis for comprehending everything you see, hear, touch, taste, and otherwise experience. Examining your paradigms is not a natural thing to do because it's a little like asking a fish to describe the fish tank in which she lives. I'm sure you can imagine that a fish isn't likely to even know she's swimming inside a tank; to the fish, her tank is simply the world she inhabits.

Your paradigms are *your* fish tank. You adopted them from your parents and society. They're neither right nor wrong, and any paradigm will remain viable until it is no longer relevant or until another, more accurate one rises to take its place.

Whether or not you've done so before, examining your paradigms thoroughly is vital to achieving your ideal body. We're about to do that right now.

> *"The important thing in science is not so much to obtain new facts as to discover new ways of thinking about them."*

William Bragg, Sr.
Physicist
Nobel Prize Winner

The two predominant paradigms that arose after the first scientific revolution were action based and machine based. Let's look more closely at how these paradigms were universally adopted by examining how they were adopted in just one area of society: the workplace.

Take, for instance, your job. You were most likely trained to do your job most efficiently and productively, and you are undoubtedly a cog in a larger operation. You depend on others to perform their job in support of your own, and others depend on you to perform your job so they can do theirs. If the people down the line from you don't get things done, you will suffer. And if you drop the ball, the people up the line from you will be affected.

Your company also probably has an organizational hierarchy through which people are managed and held accountable. You probably have a supervisor of some type who evaluates your performance and provides you with ongoing training and guidance regarding your effectiveness. You receive pay and hold a job title that is commensurate with your productivity and effectiveness. And the company you work for most likely motivates higher levels of employee productivity through promotions, which confer gains in pay and status.

These common characteristics of almost any job in our society are all byproducts of the work of Frederick Taylor, an American mechanical engineer credited with developing the modern structure of businesses. He applied the action and machine paradigms formed from the first scientific revolution in his concept of "scientific management," whereby workers are considered small parts in a larger machine (the business) and can be made more efficient through continual tinkering and experimentation by business owners and managers. This was the concept that modern, factory-based, mass-production businesses of the Industrial Revolution were built upon.

In the 1980s and '90s, America began to discover the limitations and pitfalls of our action- and machine-based business paradigms when foreign competition famously began to trump U.S. manufacturing efficiency.

These two paradigms were found lacking for the weight loss industry as well. Just as we've had to develop new paradigms for industry, so must we find new ways to move forward and realize true, healthful, and lasting weight loss.

After all, what do weight-loss experts recommend you do to lose weight? Take action! Diet and exercise – no matter how they're dressed up or restated – are what comprise all of the weight loss programs I've encountered. And these instructions are perfectly aligned with the paradigms of the *first* scientific revolution.

Stop and think about your own experiences with the diet industry. Haven't you been told that weight loss is directly linked to the actions you take (or don't take)? You're told to eat certain foods, avoid other types of foods, and engage in prescribed physical exercise. And if you don't lose weight, you're told you're <u>doing</u> something wrong. You're either eating too much or exercising too little, but either way, the fault is said to be with your *actions*. You've also been told that if you trace your actions backward, you can surely identify the core problems and issues that resulted in your unwanted weight in the first place. Take an action and receive a specific result: This is the action-based paradigm at its most logical conclusion, as seen in the modern weight loss industry.

Haven't you also been encouraged to approach losing weight from the context of the machine paradigm? You've been told that certain foods are handled in certain ways by certain parts of your body and digestive system. Thus, you've been told to change your body's "performance" by ingesting different foods, which will have predicable weight loss results for you. Additionally, you have been encouraged to get your "machine" in shape by exercising your "parts" using prescribed programs that will produce predictable weight loss results. Your overweight body is supposedly like a car in need of both repair and better fuel – this is the machine paradigm in full "gear" in the modern weight loss industry.

I know your first reaction may be to say, "But all those things are true!" and you're not incorrect. Remember, paradigms are neither "correct" nor "wrong," and these two paradigms remained until a better one came along.

So now my real question emerges: Even though you undoubtedly believe that those two paradigms are correct (because they are familiar to you and everyone believes them), **do they really serve you**? Have you ever really been able to count on them to lose and keep off unwanted weight?

> *"Science progresses best when observations force us to alter our preconceptions."*

Vera Rubin
Astronomer

I'm not asking you if you believe that eating healthy foods and getting exercise are good things to do to lose weight. I assume we all believe that, and for good reason. I am asking you if the current weight loss paradigms have actually *helped* you lose weight and get the body you truly desire. And I'm going to presume I already know your true answer to that question – otherwise why would you be reading this book?

So, by natural consequence, if the current weight loss paradigms are no longer serving you (and I believe they are not), it is time for some new ones! The good news is, the new paradigms for weight loss are based upon a science that's far more accurate and reliable than the old. Your new paradigms are modeled on the way the universe <u>actually</u> functions, on the new science of the second scientific revolution.

So let's lay the groundwork for those new paradigms right now.

Chapter Six - The Second Scientific Revolution: Quantum Physics and How it Shapes Our Thinking

"Not only is the universe stranger than we imagine, it is stranger than we <u>can</u> imagine."

Sir Arthur Eddington
Mathematician

The "new" science of Albert Einstein and the second scientific revolution, commonly referred to as quantum physics, is far more accurate than that of Newton. It has repeatedly been proven to be the most precise and accurate ever created – even by skeptics trying to disprove its theories!

Strangely enough, the science of quantum physics is actually the result of a failed (yet seminally important) experiment in 1887. Physicists Albert Michelson and Edward Morley spent a calendar year using classical physics (the science of the first scientific revolution) to calculate the speed at which the Earth traveled through space. When the year ended and they tabulated their results, Michelson and Morley revealed to the scientific community that the Earth was traveling at *zero miles per hour*!

The scientific community knew those results could not possibly be true, so a quest began to find a science that could accurately gauge and predict something like the speed of the Earth as it traveled around the Sun. They needed a science that could explain the behavior of the extremely tiny and incredibly massive components of our universe. You see, what Michelson and Morley famously stumbled upon is that classical physics is very accurate when explaining the world we see with our naked eyes, but its accuracy stops when we try to explain both the very small and very large objects that make up our universe.

Over the last hundred-plus years, quantum physics has virtually rewritten everything we thought we knew about our universe. And, as radically different as quantum physics is, perhaps even more intriguing is how accurate it has proven to be.

What follows are four of the main tenants of quantum physics.

- All matter is made up of organic, or unified, wholes that are often greater than the sum of their parts. This concept is called holism, and it is the polar opposite of the machine metaphor of the first scientific revolution.

- There is not necessarily a relationship between cause and effect. Action is not always caused by another force exerting itself.

- The observer and the observed cannot be separated. The observer's observation and expectations, literally, become a part of what is being observed. In fact, the observer and the observed may be said to be two different perspectives of the same thing.

- Systems are not linear; systems are equations whose effects are not proportional to their causes. There is a lack of logical sequence, correlation, or cohesion found in the universe where we once thought that everything was neatly and logically ordered.

Does anything about those four new fundamental rules jump out at you? What you probably noticed is the fundamental rules of the second scientific revolution are the polar opposite of the fundamental rules of the first. Remember too, that while those new rules may sound like science fiction, the science of the second scientific revolution is <u>far</u> more accurate and reliable than the classical physics you learned about in your high school science classes.

Furthermore, continued work and experimentation with quantum physics has shown that these new rules also apply to and affect the world we see with our naked eyes. They are not limited only to the tiniest and largest parts of our universe.

And here is perhaps the most vital point for consideration: If the rules from the first scientific revolution do not accurately describe how the universe operates, what does that say about the paradigms that were created from them – all those interpretations of the first scientific revolution that created the paradigms framing the world as you know it? If you answered that those paradigms might not be very accurate, you are correct.

"After you learn quantum mechanics you're never really the same again."

Steven Weinberg
Physicist
Nobel Prize Winner

This is great news! You will now be able to actually achieve the results you've always sought, because you will be armed with a plan based on how the universe <u>actually</u> works!

Chapter Seven - Old vs. New Science: A Comparison

"Anything you can do in classical physics, we can do better in quantum physics."

Daniel Kleppner
Physicist

Let's look at the new rules for how the universe really works by examining, side by side, the old science against the new.

You've read about the old science, classical physics, and how it changed the world. For almost three hundred years, the classical physics was the best and most accurate science we had – so the way we did things was almost entirely based upon it. You've also learned about the new science, quantum physics, and how different it is. Quantum physics is much more reliable and accurate than the old science and the way we do things will be almost entirely based upon it from now on.

Here are the four main tenants of the old science examined side-by-side with what the new science now tells us about how the universe really functions.

First, the old science said that each thing in the universe is made up of smaller parts with predictable functions; each thing in the universe is akin to a machine in the way its parts function together. We now know that this is not a true description of our universe. Quantum physics has taught us that a thing is actually made up of smaller whole systems that are often greater than the sum of their parts.

Second, the old science taught that for every action in our universe, there is an equal and opposite reaction. Quantum physics has now shown us, however, that this is also not true. Strange as it may sound, action is not always caused by something else exerting its force upon the object in motion.

Third, the old science told us that the observer and the thing being observed (as in a scientist conducting an experiment) are two separate things. Not true at all! Quantum physics corrects this by showing us, weird as it might sound, that the observer is an <u>active participant</u> in everything she observes and, in fact, *co-creates* what she observes through her expectations.

Finally, the old science showed us that events occur in a logical, rational, linear fashion. But (you guessed it) this is not true either. Quantum physics reveals that there is a general lack of cause-and-effect in our universe and that, in fact, logical sequence and correlation are *not at all* the foundation for systems or their outcomes.

Once again, I'd like to remind you that, although it can sound crazy, quantum physics is so accurate that many scientists now believe that, through it, we've come as close as humanly possible to deciphering exactly how the universe functions. When viewed side-by-side, quantum physics irrefutably supersedes classical physics. The new science is what we need to listen to and allow to guide us.

Chapter Eight - Why Old Science Can't Really Work for Long-Term Weight Loss

"If your model contradicts quantum mechanics, abandon it!"

Richard Feynman
Physicist
Nobel Prize Winner

I'll maintain throughout this book that *you* are not a failure; you have been failed by outdated ways of doing things, obsolete paradigms, which have severely curtailed your actual ability to achieve your weight loss goals. As you'll soon see in vivid detail, current weight loss programs, although built around solid and logical details, are destined to fail you because they are also created within the framework of old paradigms created from old science.

The old science, as you've learned, does not actually reflect how the universe really functions. So, therefore, when you are doing something that is based within the framework of those old-science paradigms, you can expect your results to be disappointing. And that, once again, has nothing to do with how hard you are working toward your goal, how much you desire to achieve your goal, nor how noble your intentions are regarding that goal. Weight loss, like any other goal you have, will remain elusively out of your reach as long as you are still taking actions within a framework which is based on the old science.

Weight loss is a billion dollar industry because of the old science. How hard should it be, truly, for the average person to achieve weight loss goals? The instructions are simple and straightforward - eating a healthier, wiser diet and getting more physical activity. So why "can't" you do that? Why does the average person have so much difficulty losing weight? Why are you and your neighbors, seemingly, getting heavier by the year?

It is not because you desire to be heavy. When was the last time a less-than-perfectly proportioned man or woman was paraded in front of us (via television, magazine, or movie)? When was the last time you were told that you looked great at your current weight, instead of being urged (overtly or subliminally) to look like the magazine cover-model, by any means necessary? You desire to be thinner than you are, for many reasons, and you are tired of the constant failure to achieve that.

The good news, as you've already read, is that the failure is not "you", it is the current paradigms of the weight loss industry. Built upon old science (which is not the most accurate and does not work). Allow me to illustrate this with just a few examples:

Aren't weight loss programs built upon the idea that you can tinker with your body's weight by manipulating and controlling its "parts" through diet and exercise? (This is from the first, inaccurate, rule of the old science which says that we are like a machine)

Aren't weight loss programs action-based? If you want to lose weight, you are told, you need to take certain specific actions like eating, or not eating, certain foods at certain times. (This is from the second, inaccurate, rule of the old science which states that actions will produce predictable and reliable results)

Aren't you told that getting fat is something that is happening "to" you, because of "outside" factors such as inactivity, improper diet, bad genes, a dysfunctional childhood, etc.? (This is from the third, inaccurate, rule of the old science which teaches that you can always find the cause of something by looking at what exerted force upon it)

Finally, aren't you taught that you can expect a logical outcome from your weight-loss efforts when you follow a weight loss program, as in "Lose 10 pounds in 10 days on the grapefruit diet!"? (This is from the fourth, inaccurate, rule of the old science which says that things happen in a logical and linear fashion)

And none of these promises materialized for you, did they? Maybe you saw the expected results temporarily, but not as you were promised. Now you know why not; the weight-loss programs were teaching you good things to do, but they were teaching them within the paradigms of the old, incorrect science of the first scientific revolution! The weight loss industry, with the best of intentions, made promises it could never deliver – because the universe doesn't really function in the way they assume it does. The old science does not work.

The deck was stacked against you from the beginning. It's as if you were trying to build a five-bedroom house with blueprints for building an equipment shed.

But now, armed with my plan, you will finally be ready to find success and feel good about your weight, your body, and food in general. You're about to become the beneficiary of new paradigms from the definitive and faithful rules of the second scientific revolution. These new rules, you're about to realize, work perfectly to facilitate losing unwanted weight and keeping it off forever.

The fundamental rules of quantum physics completely dispel the authenticity of both the action-based and the machine paradigms, the two main paradigms from the old science upon which the weight loss industry is based. The next two chapters will show you how.

Chapter Nine - New Science Fact #1: It's an Energy-Based Universe

"Reality is merely an illusion, albeit a very persistent one."

Albert Einstein
Physicist
Nobel Prize Winner

Now it's time to learn about the new paradigms that will serve as your wellspring for losing unwanted weight.

Let's begin by replacing the action-based paradigm of the first scientific revolution with one that more accurately reflects the way our universe really operates: an energy-based paradigm. Science now tells us that your actions are, quite literally, <u>not</u> the most important component for any event or circumstance.

The action-based paradigm stresses that every movement in our universe can be explained by finding the thing that has exerted itself upon that which has moved. Forces such as gravity, momentum, mass in motion, or, simply, someone or something pushing are always responsible for any movement. This is a logical explanation for movement and not only jibes with our common sense, but also meets the "naked eye" test. In fact, Isaac Newton found the idea of anything contrary to the action-based paradigm to be completely irrational and utter nonsense.

The action-based paradigm is also applied to non-physical movement such as your state of mind, your decisions, political movements, business, and philosophy. If, for example, you have a problem in your life (like unwanted weight), you have been taught that non-physical forces are probably responsible. Forces such as your upbringing, social expectations, popular culture, and the way you were parented as a child are all thought to be responsible for your problem in the action-based paradigm. Once again, this is logical to us and is generally accepted because it is logical and makes common sense.

But you don't even need the second scientific revolution to know, intuitively, that this metaphor has too many limitations when applied to your body. Your state of mind certainly appears to be context dependent. You have seen too many examples of people who are not affected by the same issues to know that a force applied to you will not always produce a predictable result.

For example, you know that many people have overweight parents yet remain quite thin and healthy. You also know that there are people who had horrible childhoods yet have not experienced unwanted weight (let alone other problems). Some have diets that you consider unhealthy, and get less exercise than you'd say is necessary, yet remain thin. While others (perhaps you) adhere to a strict diet and see little reduction in your unwanted weight. It's obvious that the same forces do not produce predictable, reliable, or consistent results when applied to different recipients.

The energy-based paradigm represents a shift away from looking at the material world (outside of you) as what is <u>causing</u> you to feel a certain way. The mantra of the energy-based paradigm is *"I'll see it when I believe it."* The science of the second scientific revolution shows us that the outside world is created by your inside world, <u>not</u> the other way around. Your internal energy creates the material world outside of you. Embracing this paradigm, as weird as it may sound to you right now, is as logical a scientific "next step" for humanity as embracing the Earth's revolution around the sun was for a person in the 17th century.

When you study the science of the second scientific revolution, you will learn that the entire universe is actually a field of energy called the quantum field. The quantum field is a non-local and unbounded energy field representing all possibilities. In layman's terms, it is everywhere all at once, it is endless and uncontained, and it can become, literally, anything. In other words, the quantum field is a field of energy from which you, me, trees, clouds, automobiles, toy soldiers, dental floss, planets, whales, etc. (literally, *everything*) are manifested and created.

All physical matter in the universe is manifested from the quantum field. This field waits, in a state of infinite possibility, for you to manifest the material world from it – which you do, either deliberately or accidentally, every second of every day you're alive. The material world does not pre-exist, awaiting your observation; you *create* the material world, through your observations, on a moment-by-moment basis.

> "Observations not only disturb what is to be measured, they produce it."

Pascual Jordan
Physicist

The scientific explanation for this is that electrons, literally, exist in a state of mere potential until they are observed. Strange as it sounds, your observation creates electrons' state, form, and location.

Yes - the second scientific revolution has clearly determined that you have created, from the quantum field, all that you see and experience. Everything you now see wasn't here waiting for you to discover it. Stop and look around your room right now. Every single thing you see and experience has been created, by <u>you</u>, from the quantum field. Even though it sounds like science fiction, it's not; if you weren't here to observe, those material objects wouldn't exist.

In fact, the most important quantum physics experiment (so important that Nobel Prize-winning physicist Richard Feynman called it "the only thing you need to know about quantum physics") shows us very clearly that you literally create the material world. The experiment is called the Double-Slit Experiment, and it uses an electron gun to fire electrons at a far wall through two slits.

"Any other situation in quantum mechanics, it
turns out, can be explained by saying,
'You remember the case of the experiment with
the two holes? It's the same thing.'"

Richard Feynman
Physicist
Nobel Prize Winner

The gist of this experiment is that the electrons fired through the double slits always take the form they are *expected* to take. The <u>observation</u> of the observer is what dictates the electron's form (whether wave or particle). And, stranger still, the electrons actually have <u>no</u> form until they are observed. They do not pre-exist in any certain form, waiting to be observed. The act of observing is what prompts them to take on any form at all!

Another way of framing this new paradigm is to think of it this way: the energy-based paradigm tells us we must switch our perspective from bottom-up to top-down. The old science said that the material world existed irrespective of you, the observer. Creation was a bottom-up process – the material world existed in a pre-determined state, awaiting your discovery.

The new, more accurate science tells us just the opposite; the material world is actually created by you, through your discovery or observations. Creation, it turns out, is a top-down process – the building blocks of all material things exist in a state of mere unrealized potential until you (the observer) turn your attention to them and command them to take a concrete and final form.

From this perhaps bizarre-sounding science of the second scientific revolution, we can construct a much more accurate, energy-based paradigm to replace the outdated action-based one. If you're not yet convinced that your actions are almost irrelevant when compared to the importance of your expectations, you soon will be.

Quantum physics shows us that we create our material world from the quantum field through our *observations*. Since the quantum field has the potential to become, literally, anything, it responds to our observations to know what to materialize as. In other words, you see and experience exactly what you *expect* to see and experience.

For example, you expected to see the chair you sat in when you entered the room, so it was waiting for you – created for you from the quantum field. You expected to experience the lamp lighting the room so you could read, so the lamp was waiting for you – also created for you from the quantum field. And so it is with every single thing you encounter, every experience you have, every moment of every day.

For the purposes of our new energy-based paradigm, let's next look at where your expectations come from. Your expectations are derived almost wholly from your beliefs; what you *believe* dictates what you *expect*. For example, if you believe (as I hope you do) that your parents love you, then that belief drives your expectations, which in turn directs the quantum field to deliver corresponding physical manifestations to you. Your parents' smiles, hugs, phone calls, notes, etc., all manifest to match your expectations (which spring from your beliefs).

Your material experiences will always match your beliefs because your beliefs drive your expectations. And your expectations will, of course, dictate what the quantum field should manifest for you.

The next logical question to complete the energy-based paradigm is this: Where do your beliefs come from? While a belief carries with it the overwhelming feeling of being "correct," you must understand that any belief you hold is only correct **for you**. Although it sometimes seems it should be, a belief is not independently correct. Nor should it be assumed to universally apply to everyone (or anyone) else. Why not? Because a belief is nothing more than something you have told yourself for so long that it has assumed that mantle for you and *you alone*!

"Observations not only disturb what has to be measured, they produce it... We compel the electron to assume a definite position... We ourselves produce the result of the experiment."

Pascual Jordan
Physicist

We can agree that most people share the same general beliefs about our world. We may not agree on the particulars like which religion is right, which political party is correct, or what television show is the best, but we do have a general, collective agreement about the way our physical world functions and the way our societies operate. We are taught what to believe (indoctrinated, if you will) about the way our physical world and our society functions primarily by our parents, television, schools, religions, government, and the popular media.

And I'm sure you can agree that, while some of the beliefs we're taught are done purposefully and overtly, many of them are conveyed to us subliminally and subtly.

My point here is not to introduce or reinforce the idea that we have been victimized by having been taught beliefs that, perhaps, don't serve us. But it is still accurate to say that you have most likely been using a system of beliefs that were *given* to you (whether you asked for them or not) and many of these beliefs, undoubtedly, do *not* serve you. You currently subscribe to beliefs that, through your expectations, create unwanted things from the quantum field and are also creating unwanted levels of bad results, like unwanted weight, in your life experience. More about that later.

For now, understand that through the energy-based paradigm we can say the physical world is not what is most "real" in the sense that it *is* completely subjective and created solely through our beliefs (and the expectations that arise from them). In other words, within this paradigm, as your beliefs change, so will your expectations, and so will your physical world. And, just as your beliefs and expectations are unique and different from mine, so too will you see and experience a different world than me. How different? That merely depends on how different are our beliefs and expectations.

Your energy is the source of the "outer" world that we have erroneously been led to believe is pre-existing, concrete, and unchanging. While you can see, touch, smell, and hear the physical world, it seems to be the most "real." But, since it is your inner energy that creates the physical world, isn't it more accurate to say that your inner energy is actually *much more real* than the physical world itself?

And the scientific fact that your outer, physical world is derived from your inner energy makes this new paradigm essential for your weight loss success. You no longer need to focus on or stress over your actions; all you need to do is learn the correct beliefs, and your unwanted weight will be a thing of the past. The world of your inner energy will set you free.

"The doctrine that the world is made up of objects whose existence is independent of human consciousness turns out to be in conflict with quantum mechanics and with facts established by experiment."

Bernard d'Espagnat
Physicist

Dr. Deepak Chopra talks about Dr. Wilder Penfield, a famous Canadian neurosurgeon whose research discovered the brain's sensory and motor cortex, among other things. During his studies of the motor cortex, having found the area of our brain where decisions are *carried out*, Dr. Penfield was said to have been excited by the prospect of one day finding the area of our brain where decisions are *made*. It may surprise you to learn that Dr. Penfield never found that part of our brain – because there is no part of our brain where decisions are made.

In fact, there is no part of your physical body where decisions are *made*. Your body, and every part of it, is an elegant tool. Perfect for *executing* decisions but not *making* them. Yet you know beyond a shadow of a doubt that you are making decisions every day. So who is making those decisions if it's not your physical body? The only possible answer must be that there is a non-physical "you" and, since this energy is making your decisions, this non-physical energy is much more "you" than your body is!

Dr. Penfield's research tells us that the real you, the one making the decisions your elegant body is carrying out, is a non-physical energy. I'll go into this concept in greater detail later, but now it's time to learn the second new paradigm that will set you free from your unwanted weight once and for all.

Chapter Ten - New Science Fact #2: It's a Holistic Universe

"Quantum physics thus reveals a basic oneness of the universe."

Erwin Schrodinger
Physicist
Nobel Prize Winner

Your body is not a machine composed of smaller parts (with predictable functions) working collectively to serve and further the larger entity. The second scientific revolution teaches us that it is more accurate to replace the machine paradigm with the holistic paradigm. Viewing your body and mind through the holistic paradigm will open doors of weight loss that had previously remained locked for you.

The machine paradigm says that a complex system can be explained by reducing it to its smallest, fundamental parts. Quantum physics shows us, however, that this is not true. Systems, as you've learned, cannot be defined so simply. In the machine paradigm, systems are fixed; that is, they remain the same in all situations. You don't need the second scientific revolution to know, intuitively, that this metaphor has too many limitations when applied to your body. Your very nature is context dependent. You have many sides and facets to your character that are drawn out by different circumstances or associations.

Sometimes a driver cutting you off in traffic will elicit a very angry response from you, while at other times it doesn't bother you the slightest bit. If the machine paradigm were truly most accurate, you would have the same response to being cut off in traffic every time.

The machine paradigm is exact and stresses a "black or white," "either/or" vision that does not work for your body or your mind. Such a paradigm offers no real role for free will. Your body is thought of as a machine whose parts are powered by external forces beyond your scope or control. For example, many people will tell you that subconscious influences from your childhood are causing you to be overweight today. Whether you currently believe this is true or not, it is an example of the machine paradigm in action, and it is too limiting.

The second scientific revolution tells us that systems aren't modeled after a machine. Instead, they're holistic. While the machine paradigm would have us deconstruct our bodies and minds, the holistic paradigm asks us to look at our bodies and minds as whole systems to better understand them. Instead of breaking down our bodies and minds into smaller parts, we look at the entire body or mind and see how their different components, often greater than the aggregate, interact and cooperate to form a whole system.

In fact, think of your body as a collection of "free agents" or whole, independent systems, just as vital individually as they are when taken as a collective (the "collective" being, of course, "you" in your entirety). These systems that make up "you" are cooperating for no known reason, but there is ample evidence that they each have their own agenda and independent actions, which are usually carried out below our level of consciousness and awareness. Some of them, such as our immune system, even offer evidence that they may have a consciousness separate from the larger "you"!

> *"The Universe begins to look more like a great thought than a machine."*

Sir James Jeans
Physicist

For example, when was the last time you commanded your heart to beat, or your lungs to breath, or your eyelids to blink? When was the last time you consciously and actively coordinated the countless nerves, muscles, tendons, etc., to work in intricate precision, allowing you to walk across the room? When did you last specifically coordinate the perfect firing of electricity through neurons across your brain's hemispheres to recall a childhood memory or your neighbor's phone number?

The machine metaphor has brainwashed

you into thinking of yourself as a machine with smaller parts and predictable functions. I hope you're realizing that this is just not so. But if you still maintain doubt or wish to cling to the old paradigm, perhaps you could benefit from what might be a shocking revelation. What follows is a true story that shows you just how independently your systems actually operate and just how much those systems' motives can sometimes trump the greater functioning of the larger system (your body)!

In the early 1990s, Dr. Candice Pert, while serving as the chief molecular biologist for the National Institutes of Health, made an amazing discovery that beautifully illustrates the concept of holism in our bodies. As opposed to a machine, where all the smaller parts' "job" is to work for the greater functions of the larger entity, Dr. Pert found amazing evidence that your body is actually a unified whole (just as the second scientific revolution predicts).

Amazing as it sounds, Dr. Pert discovered that your thoughts are real, physical things. Your thoughts, it turns out, aren't fluffy, ethereal stuff; they are tangible objects. Here's how it works.

Every thought you have, Dr. Pert found, has a unique neuropeptide associated with it, and your body, in turn, produces that unique neuropeptide every time you experience that particular thought (and the emotion associated with it). A neuropeptide is a simple, protein-based amino acid and is produced by your hypothalamus, a "control center" at the base of your brain.

Every time you have a thought, your hypothalamus "translates" that thought into billions of neuropeptides that are uniquely associated with the emotion you are experiencing because of your thought. And then your bloodstream is flooded with billions of the unique neuropeptide associated with the emotion you have just been experiencing. Your thought, translated into a neuropeptide, literally becomes a molecular messenger of emotion.

When in your bloodstream, these neuropeptides are physically assimilated by your body's cells. The neuropeptides conjoin with your cells by inserting themselves into a special receptacle on each cell's membrane – just like a key fitting into a keyhole. Each neuropeptide receptacle on a cell's membrane is specifically designed to fit just that one particular peptide and no other. So once that neuropeptide finds the right receptacle on the cell membrane, that amino acid is absorbed into the cell.

"As a man who has devoted his whole life to the most clear headed science, to the study of matter, I can tell you as a result of my research about atoms this much: There is no matter as such. All matter originates and exists only by virtue of a force which brings the particle of an atom to vibration and holds this most minute solar system of the atom together. We must assume behind this force the existence of a conscious and intelligent mind. This mind is the matrix of all matter."

Max Planck
Physicist
Nobel Prize Winner

Over time, Dr. Pert found, your cells develop more and more unique receptacles on their membranes to capture the neuropeptides to which they are most often exposed. And she also found that, over time, your cells begin to crave the neuropeptides to which they are most often exposed (and have built the unique receptacles to receive). In fact, Dr. Pert found that your cells become so accustomed to the unique neuropeptides to which they are most often exposed that they cover their membranes with nothing but receptacles for those neuropeptides. Actually shutting down other vital functions, your cells become vessels to ingest the unique neuropeptides they predominantly experience.

So your cells start "telling" your hypothalamus to produce these particular neuropeptides because they have developed an actual physical need for them. Think of a person who becomes physically addicted to a chemical, abandoning family, jobs, friends, and personal wellbeing to chase the drug, and you've got a reasonable facsimile of what happens to your cells.

One of the most sobering aspects of Dr.

Pert's findings, you're probably realizing, is that the only way your hypothalamus can produce the neuropeptides that your cells are now physically addicted to is for you to experience the emotions that will create them. And the only way your brain can experience the emotions necessary to create those neuropeptides is for it to see and experience a physical reality that will elicit those emotions.

So whether you've spent years thinking, "People don't like me," "I'm useless," and "I can't do that," or "People like me," "I'm useful," and "I can do that," you've inadvertently addicted the cells of your body, on a physical level, to the neuropeptides that your hypothalamus creates when you experience the emotions associated with those messages of either self-doubt or self-confidence. Your cells have built billions of unique receptacles for each unique neuropeptide you've predominantly exposed them to (through your emotional states). And your cells are now asking for them all day, every day. In this manner, your cells are, literally, dictating what you experience because they are controlling your emotional states. Your body has become physically addicted to certain emotional states. (Fortunately, if we have trained our cells to crave the negatively-associated neuropeptides, we can replace negative thoughts with positive ones to break the cycle and reprogram our cells to seek the neuropeptides created by thinking positive thoughts)

Not only are you *not* in charge of this process, chances are you had no idea this was even going on. Can you begin to see, through this example, that your cells are not smaller parts of a larger machine whose "job" is to serve the larger entity (your body)? Don't you agree that it's much more accurate to say that your cells, like the rest of your body, are organic wholes with independent agendas, which are greater than the sum of their parts? Your cells act like independent entities, not gears in a clock.

If your cells are calling the shots, forcing your brain to see and experience a world that will produce the emotions to which they've become addicted, isn't it easy to see that the machine paradigm in regards to your body is inaccurate? Your body's "parts" have not been behaving in reliable and predictable fashions, performing their "job" to make the larger "machine" function the way you'd most want it to, have they?

> *"Let us consider a piece of cheese. Where are its qualities? Not in the cheese, for different observers give different accounts of it. Not in ourselves, for we do not perceive them in the absence of the cheese. They are the result of the union, the seer and the seen, of subject and object."*

Robert Shea
Author

All this activity has been happening in your body without your knowledge or your consent – almost as if these systems within you have independent consciousnesses. Isn't it easy to see that, as the holistic paradigm shows, your body's smaller systems can often be called, individually, greater than the larger system they were supposed to be "serving" (under the old, machine paradigm)?

And now that you've learned the two new paradigms, based on the super accurate science of quantum physics, it's time to discover exactly how to use them on a daily basis. It's time to put these new paradigms to work for you in achieving the body of your dreams.

Part Two of Why Quantum Physicists Don't Get Fat: How to Use Quantum Physics for Long-Term Weight Loss

"We all know your idea is crazy. The question is, whether it is crazy enough."

Niels Bohr
Physicist
Nobel Prize Winner

   Part Two of <u>Why Quantum Physicists Don't Get Fat</u> is where you learn how to put this new science into action. Now begins the street-level, how-to interpretation of the science of quantum physics. The following chapters are my distillation of 15 years of research into the most modern, cutting-edge scientific knowledge available. I have researched it, digested it, and practiced it, and now I will teach you how to use it on a practical, everyday level. And I will give you the information in layman's terminology so you can easily use it to lose your unwanted weight and achieve your ideal body.

You're about to be rewarded for your investment in learning all that new science. You're about to learn exactly how to put it to use!

By the way, if you are starting here because you skipped Part One, please follow my recommendation to read Part One after you read the rest of this book. Deal?

My guess is that you're not necessarily reading this book because you want to look like the models gracing the fitness magazine covers in your grocery store. Those magazine cover photos usually involve airbrushing and/or plastic surgery anyway! Although you would probably say "yes" if a genie were granting you three wishes, I'll bet it's realistic to say you're more concerned with finally feeling good about your weight than you are with washboard abs.

If you're like most people, you just want to get off the diet merry-go-round, stop the mood swings and irritability, and feel good about yourself. You want to stop beating yourself up because you weigh too much, and you want your family and friends to be proud of you. You don't want to feel shame anymore about your failures and your wasted money. You want to look in the mirror and like what you see.

Knowing exactly how you want your ideal body to look and feel is important, and we'll explore that in greater detail later. For now, know that you're already on the way to having all those things I just mentioned.

Perhaps when you read my story in this book's preface, you decided that it wasn't tragic enough – I wasn't obese enough – and therefore, you might feel an urge to discredit this book and return to your old habits. Let me assure you that message is simply your fear and your resistance to change talking to you. Your fear will try to talk you out of these changes every step of the way, because old habits, even painful ones, are as familiar and comfortable as your favorite sweat pants.

Combat any cynicism by rephrasing an old 12-step homily: "It's not how much you weigh, it's what the unwanted weight has done to you and how it has made you feel." The bottom line is, having unwanted weight has been making you miserable, and the word "unwanted" is the primary culprit in that misery – not the specific number of pounds.

> *By 2100, our destiny is to become like the gods we once worshipped and feared. But our tools will not be magic wands and potions but the science of computers, nanotechnology, artificial intelligence, biotechnology, and most of all, the quantum theory."*

Michio Kaku
Physicist

The truth is, no one can tell you how much you should weigh and what you should look like. Some people who are living this plan began with what they considered to be a gross amount of unwanted weight, while others simply wanted to finally lose those troublesome last five pounds. Whether you have five pounds to lose or 205 pounds does not matter. You can lose it.

I've been in the prison you're in, trapped by unwanted weight. Maybe I spent too much time trying to measure up to other people's expectations for me, or perhaps I took myself too seriously, but I've certainly felt shame and guilt from carrying too much weight. I know too well the frustration that comes from continuing to gain weight despite all your best intentions and serious efforts to lose it. I understand the embarrassment of yet another failed diet and the constant flushing of money down the drain, lost in another weight loss scheme. You've been in a rut for long enough and, as I've heard it said, the only difference between a rut and a grave is the depth of the hole you're digging!

But no more. You're about to learn some simple changes that will inject any diet or exercise plan you choose with stratosphere-blasting rocket fuel! This plan has worked for me and for many others. It will work for you, too. This simple plan, if you're ready to apply yourself to it, will allow you to finally lose your unwanted weight and keep it off with relatively little suffering, stress, or strain. If you're like me and so many others, you'll find that the weight almost effortlessly goes away and stays away because you won't feel like you're "working hard" at it anymore.

Ready? Let's begin.

Chapter Eleven - You Were Born to be a Storyteller

"For as he thinketh in his heart, so is he."

Proverbs 23:7
The Bible

To begin making the full and best use of the new energy-based paradigm and the new holistic paradigm, you need to develop a cool, easy, and simple new habit. This new habit is based on the way you create your beliefs and, in turn, your expectations. And this new habit will allow you to easily create *new* beliefs that serve you and bring you into alignment with your weight-loss goals. This new habit will be your *single most important component* to implementing and using all the wonderful new tools you'll learn about in the rest of this book. It will be the foundation of your new body.

And your new habit is (drum roll please):

You're going to stop "telling it like it is" and start "telling it how you want it to be."

You'll soon see that the bad habit you currently have of "telling it like it is" is actually one of the bigger reasons you've been unable to lose your unwanted weight because of how it reinforces the old, less accurate paradigms.

To stop "telling it like it is," you will begin with a vital premise that will have great power for the creation of your new body, so it's *very important* for you to understand and embrace this idea:

No event or circumstance is inherently "good" or inherently "bad." No event or circumstance awaits you in a pre-existing state of goodness or badness. There is no such thing.

Please read the following <u>very</u> carefully: *What makes something good or bad is not the thing itself but the **story** you choose to tell yourself about it.*

The term "story" in this context simply refers to the subjective and personal meaning and value you assign to each thing, event, and circumstance in your life.

Here is an example that illustrates how your story makes something good or bad. You and a friend sit in the same movie theatre and watch the same movie at the same time. You exit the theater and proclaim, "That was the best movie ever made!" Your friend leaves the cinema and spits, "That movie was putrid; I want my money back!" Two completely divergent views of the same film.

The movie, however, is merely the movie; it was not waiting for you in a pre-existing condition of goodness or badness. <u>You</u> were the decider of whether it was a good movie or a bad movie based on your subjective judgments. It was the story you told yourself about the movie, the meaning and value you assigned to it (<u>not</u> the movie itself) that created a good movie or a bad movie for **you**.

To lay the foundation for your ideal weight, it is vital that you understand that you do the same thing with every single event or circumstance in your life. (In fact, later you'll learn just how real that movie example is) Every moment of your life, you tell a story about every single person, place, event, and circumstance, proclaiming every aspect of your life experience either good or bad.

There is nothing wrong with this; telling a story about everything (personally declaring everything to be good or bad) seems to be an integral part of the human experience. Your goal is not necessarily to *stop* telling such stories right now. All you need to do is understand that you <u>do</u> tell stories and that it's *your story* that makes things good or bad for <u>you</u>.

Here's an illustration:

An old farmer had only one horse, and one day it ran away. When the neighbors came to console the farmer over his terrible loss, the farmer said, "What makes you think it is so terrible?"

A month later, the horse came home, bringing with her two beautiful wild horses. The neighbors became excited at the farmer's good fortune. "Congratulations!" they proclaimed. "Such lovely, strong horses!" The farmer said, "What makes you think this is good fortune?"

While training the wild horses, the farmer's son was thrown from one of them and broke his leg. All the neighbors were very distressed. "Such bad luck! We are so sorry for your misfortune," the neighbors wailed. The farmer said, "What makes you think it is bad?"

A war came. Every able-bodied young man in the community was conscripted and sent into battle, where they ultimately died. The village was devastated. Only the old farmer's son, because he had a broken leg, remained behind and lived.

No one would have blamed the farmer had he ascribed each event as good or bad (as the neighbors had done). After all, any logical person could see the goodness or badness of each turn of the tale. Yet, as this story so beautifully illustrates, each event was eventually revealed to be the exact opposite of our expectations. The initial story the farmer might have told himself about each event, although logical and reasonable, <u>would have been wrong</u>!

> *"Whenever the essential nature of things is analyzed by the intellect, it must seem absurd or paradoxical. This has always been recognized by the mystics, but has become a problem in science only very recently."*

Fritjof Capra
Physicist

The old farmer's resolve to not tell a story about each event isn't supposed to make us feel like unenlightened simpletons, making judgments about everything we encounter. The point of this tale is to remind us that those stories are only *our* subjective judgments, not the unchangeable and unyielding *truth* we almost always bestow upon them! And, furthermore, the tale teaches us that our judgments are optional; whatever story you decide to tell is purely <u>your choice</u>.

Here are some examples of common life events and the logical stories you might tell about them:

- Getting an email from your friend is good, because it means she cares about you and likes you.

- Getting your gas and electric bill is bad, because the rates are too high and your limited income is being depleted.

- Getting positive results from your latest medical exam is good, because it means you're healthy.

- Your daughter's poor grades on her report card are bad, since it means she is a failure in school.

And most anyone would agree with the good or bad value you place on each event, because they're logical, reasonable, and sensible interpretations of the events described.

Yet, like the tale of the old farmer, any of these stories might be shown to be inaccurate interpretations. Perhaps the good checkup from your doctor fills you with some false confidence and you slack off on taking care of yourself – then that positive medical report might not be good, right? Perhaps your daughter's poor grades are the last straw that leads her to finally get her act together and reach her potential – then those horrible grades weren't bad, correct? Or are they? Just like the farmer's tale, I could go on and on with these illustrations of how subjective our stories of good and bad can be, repeatedly turning each story on its ear.

The point is not that we <u>shouldn't</u> be telling stories about life's events and circumstances. We will continue to do that. The point is for you to realize that your stories of good and bad are not "telling it like it is" as you've always assumed; your stories are "telling it the way you're **choosing** to tell it"! The stories you tell yourself are entirely subjective and entirely **your choice**!

And, as you're about to find out, this realization is about to make all the difference in the world for your weight loss.

Chapter Twelve - But You're Telling the Wrong Stories

"How wonderful that we've met with a paradox. Now we have hope of making some progress."

Niels Bohr
Physicist
Nobel Prize Winner

You and I tell stories that assign meaning to <u>everything</u> in our life, every moment of every day. We tell stories about all the people, places, events, and circumstances we encounter, assigning value and meaning to every single detail of our lives. Why, we're such good storytellers that we put Mother Goose to shame!

Obviously, you are reading this book because you weigh more than you want. And your unwanted weight is a direct byproduct of a specific problem you have developed with your storytelling that, when solved, will allow you to freely use your two new paradigms (energy-based and holistic) and quickly achieve your ideal body. Conversely, until you solve your storytelling problem, all the weight-loss diets, fads, gimmicks, pills, and potions in the world can't help you.

I'm about to solve this problem for you and you can then begin using your two new paradigms to lose weight quickly. Allow me to illustrate your storytelling problem through three examples. You may find these examples odd or even unsettling, but read through them carefully because they illustrate a problem you must change before you'll find true and lasting weight loss.

Let's start with an example of a, perhaps, ludicrous event with a very obvious story you'd tell about it: kicking an innocent puppy out a tenth-story window. If you surveyed everyone in your city, every person would definitively say that kicking a puppy out a window is "bad." I concur and I'm sure you do too. But that does not mean that the act of kicking a puppy out a window is inherently "bad", it means we are all telling the same story about it; we all make the same judgment and rightfully so! I wouldn't expect anyone to say, "I'm not going to call kicking a puppy out the window 'bad' because that's merely a story I'm telling myself; kicking a puppy out the window might be 'good'." Kicking a puppy out a window is bad!

And here's the most important point of this first example - because you, like everyone else, tell yourself that kicking an innocent puppy out a tenth-story window is "bad", I know you would never kick a puppy out a tenth-story window!

For our second example let's use a, perhaps, unsettling event with a less obvious story you'd tell about it: forcing someone to leave a homeless shelter where he has been staying. If you, once again, surveyed everyone in your city, you would undoubtedly get a mixed reaction of "good" and "bad". Some stories would angrily call the action "bad", as in "You're taking away his last hope and all but signing his death certificate!" While other stories might call the action decidedly "good", as in "You're making room for someone more deserving and this is probably the tough love he really needs to get motivated to change his life!" We'd probably find most of the stories falling somewhere in-between those two extremes.

In my second example, which story is the "truth"? Is it "good" or is it "bad" to force a person out of a homeless shelter where he has been staying? You already know that the correct answer to that question is that the "truth" is subjective – whether it is "good" or "bad" is all based upon, literally, whatever story you tell yourself. But, unlike the first example, when faced with a less obvious event can't you easily see that even though someone else's story might be different from yours, there is still understandable logic and reason behind their story?

This once again illustrates just how subjective, unique, and individual your story is, regarding whether a person, place, thing, event, or circumstance is "good" or "bad".

And here's the most important point of this second example: whether or not *you* would force a person to leave a homeless shelter would depend on the story you told yourself about that action. And, while I don't know you personally, I'll bet I know this about you: you *wouldn't* force a homeless person to leave a shelter if the story you told about that action made it "bad".   And, alternatively, you would *only* force him to leave if the story you told about that action made it "good."

> *"Reality is in the observations, not in the electron."*

Werner Heisenberg
Physicist
Nobel Prize Winner

Finally let's use an example of a, seemingly, innocent action that hits closer to home: eating a big, gooey, decadent, hot, fresh cinnamon roll for breakfast. What story would the people of your city tell about that action? You'd get a really mixed bag, to be sure, without nearly as many strong-feeling stories as in the first two examples. What would *your* story be? Is it "good" or is it "bad" to eat a delicious cinnamon roll for breakfast?

You might be surprised to learn that the important point of this example is <u>not</u> whether you think it's "good" or "bad" to eat a big, gooey, decadent, hot, fresh cinnamon roll for breakfast. I'll bet I already know what story you'd tell about that. The most important point about this example is that you've undoubtedly been telling yourself that eating a cinnamon roll is "bad"…and you have been <u>eating it anyway</u>! This, in a nutshell, is the storytelling problem that's played such a pivotal role in keeping your unwanted weight on you.

So let's recap. You would <u>never</u> kick a puppy out of a 10th story window because that is "bad". And you would <u>never</u> force a person out of a homeless shelter if you called that action "bad". But, on a daily basis, you <u>are</u> eating food (whether that food is a cinnamon roll or something else) that you're telling yourself is "bad" (and somehow thinking you can escape the consequences).

Eating something you call "bad" and not suffering unwanted consequences (like, of course, weight gain) would violate both of your new paradigms. And those paradigms are based upon the super-accurate, incredibly reliable science of quantum physics. You know you couldn't escape the consequences if you did the "bad" thing in the first two examples. What makes you think the consequences for this incongruence are any less severe when used with food? Hint – they *aren't* and you've been suffering from them for a while now in the form of unwanted weight!

> *"We don't see things as they are,*
> *we see them as we are."*

Anais Nin
Author

Telling yourself that something is "bad" and doing it anyway is a <u>huge</u> problem and it is, in fact, your storytelling problem. This storytelling problem is a huge part of the reason you weigh more than you'd like! Much more so then the particular foods you are (or aren't) eating. And the same is true for exercising, by the way.

By the way, I often wonder why more people don't talk about the stories you tell yourself, and the feelings they produce for you, as the most important element of any weight management program. Obviously, most people don't understand the importance of your feelings and are still stuck in the belief that the only things important are the actions you take. Perhaps some people realize, as I do, that once you learn how to do this you will stop being a customer of weight-loss products and plans because whatever diet and exercise plan you choose will work just as advertised.

After all, according to Marketdata research, Americans alone spend over $60 billion a year on weight-loss products! I hope I take a lot of money out of the hands of the weight loss industry by teaching you how to use the energy-based paradigm and the holistic paradigm to make your diet and exercise plan work like magic. Because when you're finished reading this book, you will never need to seek out the next miracle diet fad again!

I'm glad to give you an option, a way out, a ticket to freedom after you've endured a lifetime of nonstop body-image assault. You cannot turn on the television, go to a movie, read a magazine, or even get on the internet without being showered by images of bodies created through surgery and Photoshop! Razor-thin women with outlandish curves. Gorgeous men with washboard abs and steel jaws. This constant bombardment of impossibly perfect bodies has led you to tell yourself stories about how you look that not only don't serve you, they also cause you shame and pain.

I want to be clear that, because of the way you've been conditioned to tell stories about your weight, I hope you never refer to yourself as "fat," because it's an ugly word. And when you use it in your stories about yourself, you almost always feel ugly too.

In fact, try an experiment right now. Say out loud, "I am fat." How did that feel? Now say out loud, "I have unwanted weight." If you're like me, saying "unwanted weight" felt a lot better than saying "fat."

Why are these words important? Because, just as the stories themselves are important, the words you use to tell your stories are meaningful and carry a punch. You'll learn more about their importance later. For now, here's why I never want you to refer to yourself as fat. You are <u>not</u> fat! Fat is not your state of being. Fat does not define you as a human being, and it is not *what* you are.

Go back to the two statements in our experiment. Could you recognize the difference between "I am fat" and "I have unwanted weight"? I'll underline the words that make those two statements as different as night and day:

"I <u>am</u> fat."

"I <u>have</u> unwanted weight."

The first statement says that "fat" is *who you are*; the second statement says that you are merely *experiencing* unwanted weight but that the unwanted weight is <u>not</u> *who you are*.

Just as I want you to start telling stories that serve you, I want you to use *words* that serve you by uplifting and enhancing you, not degrading you. In this book, you're learning exactly how to do that.

It's time for you to start telling yourself new stories about food, new stories about moving, and new stories about your body. And, in fact, your ideal weight will only be achieved when you are telling these new stories and feeling better about eating, moving, and accepting yourself *right where you are.* No longer do you have to repeat and believe those stories that hurt you and keep you imprisoned in unwanted weight!

"Creation is always happening. Every time an individual has a thought, or a prolonged, chronic way of thinking, they're in the creation process. Something is going to manifest out of those thoughts"

Michael Beckwith
Theologian

You see, your beliefs are not the "carved in stone" *monuments of truth* you've built them into. Your beliefs are merely the stories you've told yourself long enough that they have become your truths. That's right: Your beliefs are true for *you* simply because you've told yourself the stories so many times. And by telling yourself new stories, you will, slowly but surely, create new beliefs for yourself. Building new beliefs is like building a house; you do it one brick (or, in this case, one story) at a time.

Solving this storytelling problem is your key to using your two new paradigms and to achieving and maintaining your ideal weight. Even for achieving many other things in life that have been eluding you. And solving that problem is what you're about to start doing!

Chapter Thirteen - The Big Secret to Losing Weight (or How to Tell the Right Stories)

"We are tiny patches of the universe looking at itself and building itself."

John Wheeler
Physicist

I had been on a ton of diets as my spare tire grew bigger and bigger during my 20s. If a friend told me about a diet or I saw it in a magazine headline, I probably tried it! And I worked hard at it too. Remember the no-fat diet? I ate zero fat grams…and still I eventually went back to gaining weight. I went through spells where I worked out like a madman. Of course, I also tried skipping meals all the time. I drank shakes, ate "program" food, and counted points. One time, I ate nothing but grapefruits for two days.

Nothing worked; I was still getting heavier!

And I'm sure you have a similar story. If information, good intentions, and hard work made you thin, you'd be walking a runway in Paris right now! However, there is a secret to losing and keeping off unwanted weight, and it's not a diet and it's not exercise.

Once you know this secret, you'll be able to adopt a lifestyle that will enable you to attain your ideal weight and stay there with very little effort at all. Knowing this secret will also allow you to make full and effective use of your two new paradigms. With practice, you're going to feel like your weight drops off in your sleep.

The secret? Attaining your ideal weight is *not* about what you do or don't do; attaining your ideal weight is all about how you <u>feel</u>. Diets fail you because they are about action and they treat your body like it's a machine. And exercise regimens fail you for the same reasons. Attaining your ideal weight, and keeping it, is not about the actions you take – it is about your feelings!

And learning to pay attention to your feelings will help you employ your two new paradigms for incredible weight loss.

I have explained that your beliefs create your expectations, and that your expectations create your physical experiences. Your beliefs are the internal energy that you will now learn to change and, when changed, will create a new, holistic reality for your body. And your feelings will play an invaluable role in the creation of your new body, because they serve as the "thermometers" of your beliefs.

Thermometers are pretty handy tools for knowing whether your body has a fever or not, aren't they? Well, your feelings are your built-in thermometers for your state of being, because they tell you if your beliefs are in congruence with your desires. What a great untapped asset!

In other words, your feelings tell you exactly what your current beliefs about something are. Feel good about something? That is your best sign that your current belief about that is a positive one and is aligned with your desired outcomes. And the opposite is also true. When you feel bad about something you can be pretty sure you hold a current belief about that thing that is negative and not aligned with your desired outcomes.

This information takes on added vitality when you remember that quantum physics teaches you that your beliefs create your expectations and your expectations create your reality. So pay attention to your feelings! They are letting you know what your beliefs are.

Does the importance of paying attention to your feelings mean that diet and exercise are unimportant to the attainment of your ideal weight and keeping it? Not at all. Diet and exercise are <u>great things</u>! It's just that, contrary to what you've been taught, diet and exercise are of *secondary* importance. How you <u>feel</u> about them is actually more important than what you are doing with either one.

Let me explain what I'm talking about and further illustrate how you can use the science of quantum physics in your everyday life.

The energy-based paradigm tells us that when you focus on what you don't want or upon negative goals, you not only feel bad, but you also get more of those very things you're focused on. What you focus on is what grows! In other words, when you focus on being fat and the weight you haven't lost yet, you will only get heavier and have more weight to lose. I know this is a cruel irony, but people who feel good about their diet and exercise can actually eat almost anything (with some moderation, of course)! But if you feel bad about what you're eating, you can practically eat only watercress sandwiches and still gain weight!

> *"The paradox is only a conflict between reality and your feeling what reality ought to be."*

Richard Feynman
Physicist
Nobel Prize Winner

You've been taking a lot of good actions designed to lose weight, but you've continued to gain weight simply because the stories you tell yourself are about your being fat, your needing to lose weight, and your not being successful at it.

It ultimately comes down to this: When you constantly eat and tell yourself some version of, "I shouldn't eat this" (or "I don't *want* to eat this," when dealing with healthier food), you're always going to feel bad and gain weight. When you exercise and tell yourself, "I <u>have</u> to do this even though I *don't want to*," you're always going to feel bad and not lose the weight you want to from your efforts. In both of these examples, because your focus was on what you <u>don't want</u>, you've gotten the results the energy-based paradigm teaches you to expect. That is, you've continued to gain weight and you've not been successful at losing it.

Your failure makes you feel even worse about yourself, which makes you feel even more negative about your eating plan and exercise. Do you see the horrible, self-defeating, self-perpetuating pattern here?

This pattern has taken you to the point where eating and exercising, two wonderful, beautiful, necessary actions for any human being, have become your enemies!

If you have unwanted weight, you tell yourself stories about food and exercise that do not serve you and are not aligned with your desires. In fact, you tell yourself stories about food and exercise that actually hurt you and keep weight on you!

If any of this sounds silly to you, then one of two things must be true: either you don't have unwanted weight (and if that's true, why are reading this book?) or you have not had enough pain to be *willing* to try something new (even though this new thing is the most accurate foundation for weight loss available) to lose your unwanted weight. Either perspective is, of course, okay for you to have. Even if you have unwanted weight and aren't ready to lose it, you may be right where you're supposed to be, and I hope you save this book for another time when you *are* ready.

But for those of you still with me, we're about to take this to another level.

Telling new stories about eating and moving is important because quantum physics, your two new paradigms, and your own experience have taught you that the stories you tell yourself usually come true. If you tell yourself that the food you're eating is bad for you, the food <u>will</u> be bad for you. The result? You will continue to gain more pounds. If you

tell yourself that exercise is bad, the exercise will
be bad for you and you <u>will</u> suffer while doing it.
The result? You will continue to gain more
pounds.

> *"As careful attention shows, thought itself*
> *is in an actual process of movement. That*
> *is to say, one can feel a sense of flow in*
> *the stream of consciousness not dissimilar*
> *to the sense of flow in the movement of*
> *matter in general. May not thought*
> *itself thus be a part of reality as a whole?"*

David Bohm
Physicist
Nobel Prize Winner

Perhaps worst of all, when you're on a diet
within the old paradigms, you're focused upon a
<u>don't-want</u> (your weight) and you'll always be
doomed to fail because you're focused on the bad
thing. The same is true of exercising to lose

weight. If you're focused on a <u>don't-want</u> (your weight), you're doomed to fail there, too.

But, don't worry, I'm about to teach you how to retrain your thought process and grow new beliefs that will <u>serve</u> you! These new beliefs and the new expectations that will spring forth from them will have you at your ideal weight a lot sooner than you ever thought possible.

Chapter Fourteen - Putting It into Play: Your Two-Part Plan for Your Ideal Body

"Science is a way of thinking much more than it is a body of knowledge."

Carl Sagan
Scientist

Some of what you learn from here on out may sound like some feel-good philosophy or timeworn homily. But rest assured. Everything you'll learn is designed to engage the amazing science of the second scientific revolution. Everything you will learn is important to follow *exactly as written,* and it all really works to achieve your ideal body because it will teach you how to use your two new paradigms of an energy-based and holistic universe.

Achieving and maintaining your ideal body will be achieved by learning to tell yourself new stories about two things: diet and exercise. This two-step plan is all you need to inject any diet or exercise plan with rocket fuel. It's just that simple. And because it's best to keep things as simple as possible, let's now call "diet" what it really is: eating. And let's call "exercise" what it really is: moving. So all you really have to do to achieve your ideal weight and keep it is eat and move!

I'm going to teach you how to eat and move through the filter of your feelings so that any diet and exercise plan you might choose begins to work for you like magic. You're going to learn to tell yourself different stories about eating and moving – stories that feel good and serve you, rather than the familiar, bad stories you know all too well. When you choose to eat a luscious piece of chocolate cake, for example, instead of telling yourself, "I shouldn't eat this," you're going to be saying, "I can eat this and I'm going to love every bite of it!" Your body will begin changing immediately as you start telling yourself these new stories. And now I'll show you exactly how to get started.

Chapter Fifteen - How to Eat

"Science is piecemeal revelation."

Oliver Wendell Holmes
Physician

I have the simplest rule imaginable for your eating. And it is also the *only* rule for eating: *To achieve your ideal weight and keep it, don't eat anything <u>unless you honestly feel good about it</u>. Period. No deviation. No exceptions.*

Sound too easy? Perhaps, it's simple, but it's not so easy to carry out – at least not at first.

Eating only when you feel good about it ensures many things, primarily that you are telling yourself good stories about the food you are eating and about your self-worth. And it not only ensures you will only eat food that you feel good about, it also ensures that you will always do whatever is necessary to feel good about any food you eat. When you start practicing this rule, your body and your life will begin transforming immediately.

A word of caution, though! Don't be tricked into continuing to tell yourself the wrong food stories that you've told in the past. You know the ones: "Eat that cake; you've earned it. It's delicious. One piece isn't going to kill you. You deserve it, for goodness sake! You can start being good tomorrow." Then you begin to consume the cake and the story quickly changes to some version of: "Why are you eating this? You shouldn't eat this! No wonder you're fat!" Then you finish the cake and, if you're like most, your story might even become self-abusive, "You have no self-control! You should be ashamed of yourself!"

And you look in the mirror after telling yourself these bad-feeling stories and you see an even more defeated person. You know all too well that your shame only makes it that much easier to fall for those bad food stories again the next time. Such stories repeat again and again, and they're counterproductive to your weight-loss efforts.

Whether your stories are worse than my examples or not as bad, you're definitely telling yourself stories that don't serve you. They're hurtful, and they keep you imprisoned by your weight.

Recognizing these bad stories takes practice, and the longer you've been telling yourself these stories, the more practice it may take to identify them. So be as patient with *yourself* as you're being diligent about your eating!

Truly feeling good about your food will never lead you to beat yourself up afterward.

How will you know if you *really* feel good about food and are not being tricked by your old, entrapping, and bad-feeling food stories? You'll learn to listen, <u>really</u> <u>listen</u>, to your gut. I'll give you some tools to help you do this later, but for now understand that feeling good about your food is mostly about feeling gratitude and joy. When you eat, you're doing one of the most loving things you can ever do for your body! When you feel real, genuine gratitude and joy in consuming your food (and you still feel that way afterward), you *are* feeling good about it.

Of course, there will be some food that will take you a long time to ever feel good enough about to eat. Desserts and sweets, for example, will probably challenge you for quite a while – and for good reason. Like fried foods and fast food in general, desserts are usually full of things that don't nourish and enrich your body. Remember, there is no rule that you *can't* eat such foods, but it's very difficult to actually feel good about eating some things, so for now you might not even want to try.

For example, I have never been able to feel good about eating pancakes. I have no idea why, nor do I particularly care, but even after 15 years I just can't eat them and feel good. So I very rarely eat pancakes. If you have foods like that, don't sweat it. Just avoid them.

*"Be careful how you think; your life
is shaped by your thoughts."*

Proverbs 4:23
The Bible

While there are no preset lists of foods to either eat or avoid, it will undoubtedly behoove you to find foods you can eat and feel good about. Foods such as fresh fruit, vegetables, smaller portions, whole grain, less fat, less sugar, low carbs, etc., will be much easier to feel good about eating. In fact, these types of foods may be the only foods you'll feel good about eating for a while. Why? Because that's what we've been taught (right or wrong).

Also remember that you can choose how you feel about any food. You are in control of the story you tell yourself about it. If you're like me, you'll grow to feel good about lots of healthy foods you might not have enjoyed before now.

This might be a good time for you to make an appointment with a trusted physician, nurse practitioner, and/or dietician to have a thorough conversation about food. Aside from following a specific diet, getting solid advice from a trusted professional may be very helpful as you begin the process of discerning which foods you can feel good about eating. This kind of input is a bit like adjusting your compass before setting sail. It's always good to feel confident about the direction you're traveling, and it helps that confidence to get advice from someone you trust!

And don't worry too much about not being able to eat your old favorites ever again; the more practice you get telling yourself your new stories about food, the greater variety of food you'll be able enjoy and feel good about. The more you tell yourself stories about being grateful, about being joyous, and about nourishing your body, the better you'll be able to really, honestly feel good about consuming more foods you used to beat yourself up for eating.

Take heart: I love a good bowl of ice cream or a doughnut! They taste delicious! And because I almost always eat those kinds of foods <u>only</u> when I feel good about them (which I used to <u>not</u> be able to do at all), I maintain my ideal weight with what feels like not much effort at all!

I'm confident that, with practice, you'll get there too. Especially when you combine your new eating stories with the next secret – how to move.

Chapter Sixteen - How to Move

"When you visualize, then you materialize. If you've been there in the mind you'll go there in the body."

Dr. Denis Waitley
Psychologist

I think you're ready for the challenge, so I've doubled-up the rules on you! Where eating has only one rule, moving has two.

Moving Rule #1: Move every day as often as you can.

Moving Rule #2: Feel good about your movement.

Just as with eating, you've probably been telling yourself bad-feeling stories about moving for quite a while. Perhaps you see moving as stressful, painful, hard work. Maybe you were forced to do it at some point and now you're resentful about having to move your body. Or you could just be following your habit of sitting a lot and being a passive observer of life. Whatever your current stories about moving are, you're going to find it's a lot simpler than you imagined to get up off that bench and join the game!

Moving every day as often as you can is a relatively simple rule. If you're ready, able, and willing to start jogging, lifting weights, doing yoga, and/or using exercise machines, good for you! If you're not, however, don't fret. You don't have to engage in that type of movement right now to follow this rule.

Moving every day as often as possible is as simple as walking up the stairs instead of using the elevator or the escalator. Moving is as straightforward as walking down the airport hallway rather than using the moving sidewalk. It's about using a push mower instead of a riding one (or not using the self-propel option on the push mower). If you will simply walk the three blocks to the coffee shop instead of drive, guess what? You're following this rule.

See how easy it is to move every day as often as possible? You can follow this rule by always choosing the most labor-intensive option available when you do anything or go anywhere. And if you start with the easy tasks I just mentioned, you'll soon find yourself inspired to begin doing things like taking a walk for the sole purpose of moving your body. Then, perhaps, riding your bike, practicing yoga, or jogging. You don't need to perform any particular type of movement until you, yourself, feel inspired to do so.

And even if you are at a point that you can walk, bike ride, lift weights, do yoga, use an exercise machine, etc., I <u>still</u> want you to find the most labor-intensive option available when you do it.

"What really matters for me is … the more Active role of the observer in quantum physics … According to quantum physics the observer has indeed a new relation to the physical events around him in comparison with the classical observer, who is merely a spectator."

Wolfgang Pauli
Physicist
Nobel Prize Winner

The second movement rule, feel good about your movement, is a must. This rule addresses your long-standing bad feelings about moving, which have contributed greatly to your current unwanted weight. Feeling good about your movement, you'll find, is all about the stories you tell and the attitude your stories engender. You'll find that movement is almost always within the realm of your control to feel good about.

In order to feel good about your movement, your stories about movement need to change. And this, you'll find, is easy to do and, with practice, will become second nature in no time. To begin, here is a list of phrases you should never utter again, followed by the phrases you should replace them with immediately. Use these phrases liberally throughout your day and, especially, as you practice moving as often as possible.

Replace this story	**With this story**
"I <u>have</u> to do this."	"I <u>get</u> to do this."

"I don't want to do this."	"Thank you for this opportunity to move my precious body."
"Oh no, two more flights to go."	"Oh no, <u>only</u> two more flights to go!"
"Darn it!"	"Thank you!"
"This doesn't feel good."	"Any pain I feel is only temporary and will lessen over time."
"I can't do this."	"I only need to do my best and *my best is good enough*."

And say this any time you are moving your body: "I'm so grateful for this opportunity to move my amazing body today and for this chance to feel even better about my body."

These phrases will, literally, transform your movement. And you'll create many other phrases that are unique and work well for you. They will all become the cornerstones of the stories you tell yourself about moving, and you will soon notice that you feel uplifted and grateful when thoughts of moving enter your mind and when you are anticipating the opportunity to move. The way you feel about moving is, after all, the most important part of it and always trumps action alone.

There are, however, a couple things I recommend you do to help yourself tell good stories about moving. First I encourage you to make movement fun; make moving a game. Give yourself permission to make up silly games (and keep them to yourself, if you wish). You might find, as I do, that it's fun to flex different muscles when I'm moving, to pretend I'm a member of the US (Over 40!) Soccer Team (so I'd better get in shape to help my country!), to see how many people I can wave and smile at each time I'm outside moving, to move in the company of good friends, and to plot courses for my movement that take me past houses and/or landmarks I like to see. All these games, and more, keep me encouraged and uplifted when I move; they keep movement from being a chore and "hard work" (even when I decide to push my body).

You can try my games, but I'm confident you'll also find your own games if you're open to it. As my Father, Dr. Kuhn, teaches, having an attitude and openness towards fun will almost always guarantee you'll find it. And the more fun you can have while moving your body, the better feeling the stories you'll tell about it will be. Before long, you'll be inspired to try things you never imagined, like yoga or kayaking, all because you've made a commitment to have fun with movement.

> *"The influence of modern physics goes beyond technology. It extends to the realm of thought and culture where it has led to a deep revision in man's conception of the universe and his relation to it."*

Fritjof Capra
Physicist

The second thing I recommend you do in addition to telling yourself good stories about moving is to stay focused only on *today*. Don't think about the movement you *didn't* do yesterday (or yesteryear). Instead, focus on the movement you're doing today. Trying to "make up" for movement you haven't been doing is impossible and won't produce good-feeling stories about moving. All you need to do is move as much as you can today and only today. However much you move today is enough! In fact, pat yourself on the back, big time, for any movement you do today! A friend who does water aerobics three times a week at the YMCA told me that her instructor concludes each class by having the students wrap their arms around their shoulders and give themselves a pat on the back. What a nice self-affirmation after a good workout!

As with eating, this might be a good time to consult with a physician, nurse, or certified trainer about safe movement.

And as with your eating, remember to be easy with yourself about your movement. Yes, I do expect you to move as much as possible each day and I do expect you to feel good about your movement as you do it. But my expectation for you is progress, not perfection. We all experience ups and downs. Bad days will come, illness will intrude, and energy will be low sometimes. These things are okay. Do not beat yourself up for falling shy and do not try to "make up" for the lost movement later. I hereby give you permission to make mistakes. Doing your best today is *all* you ever need to do!

Trust that, over time, your attitude will "shape up" in tandem with your body and you will get the inspiration to do whatever is necessary at just the right time.

And now it's time to share my tried-and-true six indispensable tools for telling the best stories to shape and maintain your ideal body.

Chapter Seventeen - Six Indispensable Tools for Shaping and Maintaining Your Ideal Body

"There are only two ways to live your life. One is as though nothing is a miracle. The other is as if everything is."

Albert Einstein

Physicist

Nobel Prize Winner

You've undoubtedly already started losing your unwanted weight and begun feeling differently about your body by practicing the three simple rules you've learned about food and movement. You're only eating what you feel good about eating. You're moving as much as possible every day. And, while moving, you're feeling good about your movement.

Congratulations! As you now know, the results of these changes are real and they manifest almost immediately.

In addition to those three rules, I want to teach you some tools you can use that will make it even easier for you to lose your unwanted weight and keep it off for the rest of your life. These tools amplify the results you'll see from good eating and moving, making them more dramatic, impactful, and powerful. They will feel like you've replaced a rusty old handsaw with a heavy-duty chainsaw.

These tools, like the three rules for your eating and moving, will become second nature and habitual with practice. At first, like the three rules, they may feel like a radical departure from the way you've always conducted yourself. But, even if they feel strange, trust that they will be of great help to you and apply yourself to them as thoroughly as you're able. They have been gleaned from years of studying with experts in self-growth like my father, Dr. Kuhn, Dr. Deepak Chopra, Dr. Wayne Dyer, and many others.

I suggest you take each one of these six tools and focus on that tool for a week. Every month and a half you'll have cycled through all of them and, after a year, you'll have spent eight weeks focused on each tool. If you commit yourself to that schedule, while you practice the three simple rules of eating and moving, you won't even recognize yourself after the year is over! And, in fact, you'll see amazing changes in your body (and your attitude) long before the year is up.

As with the three simple rules for eating and moving, take it easy on yourself with these six tools. Your goal is to practice them every day, as often as possible. But definitely do not beat up on yourself if you forget to practice them or if you feel like you're not getting as much from them as you should. There is no expectation of mastery for these six tools. There is no time you'll be able to say, "I'm finished; I now practice them perfectly!" Your goal is simply to get better and better at using them with each passing day, and also to experience the way your life improves as you practice.

Tool #1: Always Tell the Best Story Possible

"The real voyage of discovery consists not in seeking new lands but seeing with new eyes."

Marcel Proust

Author

One thing that quantum science has taught us, beyond a shadow of a doubt, is that there is no such thing as a detached observer. We all grew up with the image of a scientist watching an experiment and recording the data. But quantum physics tells us that this is impossible, because the observer acts as a direct participant in all that's being observed, which creates outcomes affected by the observer's expectations.

There are quantum experiments, with accuracy within 1/100 of a decimal point, showing us that the observer's expectations create the physical form that matter takes. Your expectations, literally, create the physical world around you. I realize this may be a huge shift for you and, perhaps, even hard for you to believe, but I assure you that quantum physics proves this definitively. So, even if you struggle to believe this data, allow me to help you begin using it to not only shed unwanted weight and keep it off, but also improve many other aspects of your life.

Telling yourself the best story possible is a phenomenal way to apply the discoveries of quantum physics, and it is a great tool for losing unwanted weight. You already know that you tell stories about every person, place, thing, and circumstance in your life. You assign meaning to them, you designate each of them as being good or bad. There is nothing wrong with you telling these stories – it seems that's what you were born to do.

And, although you can choose what story you tell most of the time (especially with practice), you are not supposed to be able to magically make any person, place, thing, and circumstance good just because you have the freedom of choice. Certainly, masters of thought can transcend placing value and judgment upon life's events, but you and I are probably not going to be able to devote the energy, study, and practice necessary to join them.

This is why I am telling you to tell the "best story *possible*" at all times and not telling you to "always tell a good story."

When you discover that your beloved pet dog has been killed by an automobile, for example, you are not expected to be able to tell a story that makes that event good. For you, and almost every human, those types of life events are sad, frustrating, maddening, anguishing, and gut-wrenching. If we're fully invested in our lives, such tragedy is supposed to feel that way.

However, if you're like most people, you can also think of many times when you interpreted fairly innocuous events as "bad." Not getting a phone call returned, someone breaking up with you, not getting a job, losing your electricity, or having a friend move away are all examples of things that you might've judged bad and told a bad-feeling story about when they occurred. Yet, with the passing of time, retrospect shows you that some of these things were actually good (or, at least, not nearly as bad as you judged them when they happened).

So remember this important tool each day and practice it as often as possible. Tell the best possible *believable* story for each person, place, thing, and circumstance you encounter. This means that you will not rush to label anything bad and, wherever possible, you will find a way to tell a good story about it. For example, when you don't get the job you wanted, instead of saying, "This is horrible; I never get what I want!" you can tell this story: "This must not have been the job I'm supposed to get. Perhaps my best job is still out there and is still waiting for me!"

Remember my movie example from earlier in the book? Now that you understand the truth behind the stories you tell and your choices regarding those stories, I hope you can see that your life is actually just like a movie. Except in this movie you are not only the star and the director, you are the one writing the script!

If you step on the scale and find, to your surprise, that you have gained two pounds, you don't have to tell a bad-feeling story and say, "I'm a failure!" Instead you can choose a better feeling story like, "Although I am disappointed that I've gained two pounds instead of losing weight like I hoped, I can use my disappointment to motivate me tomorrow. In that way, these two pounds might end up being a blessing." But even if your story is not quite as good feeling as my examples, all you need to do, at any time, is simply tell the best possible story you can muster.

When a truly unwanted tragedy strikes, like your dog dying, of course the best possible story you can tell, at that moment, might be, "This sucks!" That's okay; I *never* want you to pretend like you're not unhappy. If that's your best possible story (and I'm sure it would be for me, too) then you've done all you can and you've still used this tool to your fullest. Over the course of time, the story you can tell about such an emotional event will grow better and better.

And there is another reason that this tool is called "Always Tell the Best Story <u>Possible</u>" instead of "Always Tell a Good Story." It's because you should tell a story you'll *believe*. Believing your story is of paramount importance. For example, if you get fired from your job and, moments later, you try to tell yourself, "This doesn't suck! This is awesome! I'm so glad this happened!" I doubt you could really believe that under almost any circumstances. But perhaps you might be able to believe a story like, "This sucks! But I can choose to believe that, in the long run, I'll be okay and might even look back on this as a blessing." That feels better and remains believable, doesn't it? Or maybe the best story you can tell yourself is, "This sucks! It won't feel bad forever, but it sure does suck right now!" That's still believable and it certainly feels better than, "I'm a failure! My life is ruined. Things never work out for me!"

Here is a wonderful story that illustrates how one man told the best possible stories, even about tragic events, and how it changed his life for the better:

An African king had a close friend who had the habit of remarking, "This is good" about every occurrence in life, no matter what it was.

One day, the king and his friend were out hunting. The king's friend loaded a gun and handed it to the king. But, alas, he loaded it wrong. And when the king fired it, his thumb was blown off.

"This is good!" exclaimed his friend.

The horrified and bleeding king was furious. "How can you say this is good? This is obviously horrible!" he shouted.

The king put his friend in jail.

About a year later, the king went hunting by himself. Cannibals captured him and took him to their village. They tied his hands, stacked some wood, set up a stake, and bound him to it. As they started to set fire to the wood, they noticed that the king was missing a thumb. Being superstitious, they never ate anyone who was less than whole. They untied the king and sent him on his way.

Full of remorse, the king rushed to the prison to release his friend.

"You were right, it was good," the king said.

The king told his friend how the missing thumb saved his life, adding, "I feel so sad that I locked you in jail. That was such a bad thing to do."

"No! This is good!" responded his delighted friend.

"Oh, how could that be good, my friend? I did a terrible thing to you."

"It is good," said his friend, "because if I hadn't been in jail I would have been hunting with you and they would have eaten <u>me</u>!"

As quantum physics shows us, by looking for ways to feel as good as possible about people, places, things, and circumstances in your life, you are creating even more good in your life by telling yourself the best story possible.

As you practice telling the best story you can, you will not only continue shedding any unwanted weight and keep it off, but you will also begin to see more good in everything you do. This is how the universe operates: It delivers what you expect to see rather than what you hope to see.

Tool #2: Focus on the Feelings You Want, Not the Pounds You Want to Lose

"In these days, a man who says a thing cannot be done is quite apt to be interrupted by some idiot doing it."

Elbert Green Hubbard
Author

One of the surest and fastest ways to bring anything into your experience, including the loss of unwanted weight, is to concentrate on the feelings you'll have *when you achieve your goal.*

Focusing on the goal, itself, usually brings up feelings of "Why isn't it here yet?" So make it your business to focus on the <u>feeling</u> you expect that goal to give you. Of course, right now, your goal is to lose your unwanted weight and keep it off, but this tool works for anything in life you want.

Once again, this tool is a liberal application of something quantum physics has taught us: In the physical world, like attracts like. You've heard this principal discussed as the "law of attraction". I can assure you the law of attraction is essentially real, and its underpinnings are found in the realm of science.

For our physical, human experience, we should pay attention to our feelings, for it is our feelings that tell us what we're attracting and bringing into our experience. Have you ever struck a tuning fork and heard how it vibrates? You probably know that a vibrating tuning fork will cause any other tuning fork, tuned to the same pitch, to begin vibrating in unison with it.

Think of your feelings as a tuning fork and think of the people, places, things, and experiences of your life as millions of tuning forks filling up the entire universe. When you ring your tuning fork, when you feel your feelings, all the tuning forks (the people, places, things, and experiences) that are tuned the same will begin to ring also. This is a literal explanation of the law of attraction in action.

As with the first tool, this one presents you with what might be a huge shift and might also be challenging for you to believe. But if you're willing to try this tool, I believe you'll find enough amazing results that you'll soon be an unqualified convert.

To start using this tool right away, create a list of good feelings you expect to have when you achieve your desired weight. (If it helps, revisit the list of feelings in my preface to this book) Maybe your list has some more personal feelings as well. Whatever your list consists of, it will become even more powerful if you write it down on a piece of paper. And try to feel those feelings, right now, as you write them down.

Do not wait until something happens to "make" you feel these feelings; feel them for no "outside" reason at all! Try to feel them as often as possible each day, no matter what is going on around you. Give yourself permission to feel them right now and bask in their glow! To remind yourself, jot each list item on a small notepad and stick copies on your mirror, your desk at work, your computer screen, and your car dashboard.

Why will this work for you? If you're like most people, you are in the habit of focusing on what you want – but on the fact that it is not there yet. If you focus on the weight you want to lose and the weight loss hasn't happened yet, you're constantly focused on some version of "Where is my weight loss? It's not here. I wish I would lose the weight!"

And because like attracts like in our universe, you get what you focus on: "It's not here yet." Focusing on the feelings you want, <u>by feeling those feelings as often as possible</u>, will bring dramatic results.

By feeling the fantastic feelings you previously put off feeling, you are ringing your tuning fork at a new and different frequency, one that sounds like, "I am light, I am sexy, I am free, I am healthy, etc." And now, automatically, other tuning forks tuned to the same frequency will begin to vibrate in unison with you. Like-tuned people, places, things, and experiences will begin to manifest and come to you. They will all be attracted to your feeling vibrations. It is the law of our universe.

Remember the old saying "I'll believe it when I see it?" You're going to find out that the correct way to state it is "I'll see it when I believe it." Because, by feeling the feelings of your success <u>before</u> the success is in your material reality, the universe will automatically begin bringing to you those people, places, things, and experiences that will make that success manifest in your material reality. It will feel like magic if you really make an effort to feel those feelings you listed as often as possible each day.

Take it easy on yourself as you practice this, though. You've spent your entire life looking at "what is" and focusing on the absence of the things you desire, saying, "Where is it?" Don't beat up on yourself when you lapse back into your old habits; just take that as a reminder that you're not perfect yet (and aren't supposed to be) and start feeling your desired feelings again.

Tool #3: Meditate for 15 Minutes Each Day

"What things soever you desire, when you pray, believe that you receive them, and you shall have them."

Mark 11:24
The Bible

Who are you? I can tell you, with almost complete certainty, who you are *not*. You are <u>not</u> your brain – even though your brain wants so badly to be who you are. And, in fact, your brain's struggle to be who you are has caused a lot of problems for you – including your unwanted weight. You're about to get on the path to remedying those problems right now.

What I'm calling your brain, some refer to as your ego. Whichever term you use, if you're like most people you have spent your life listening to your brain's constant and incessant dialogue and you have come to believe that dialogue is "you." Your brain is pretty persuasive, and just about every human being falls for its act, so don't feel bad about getting duped.

However, for your brain to assume the identity of "who you are," your brain has to rely heavily upon fear and anger. You see, your brain has to get you to stay focused upon the future (obsessed about what *might* happen) and the past (obsessively rehashing everything that *has* happened and ruminating upon why it was good or bad). That is because your brain knows that who you *really* are can only be found <u>in the present moment</u>. So, in turn, your brain can only keep its identity as who you are by getting you *out* of the present moment.

Today, science understands that your brain is an elegant tool, more powerful and advanced than anything we can imagine. Yet it is only a tool, just like your heart, lungs, muscles, or nervous system. You make decisions every day. You decide to walk the stairs instead of taking the escalator, you decide to eat an apple instead of a cupcake, you decide to scratch your ear, you decide to turn left, etc. Your brain facilitates those decisions through your motor and sensory cortexes, but it does not *make* any decisions!

That's right, modern science has yet to find *any* part of your brain where decisions *are made*, only where they are carried out. Yet there is no doubt that there exists a "you" who is making decisions for your brain (and the rest of your body) to execute. This means that the real "you," the "you" that <u>decides</u>, is a non-physical energy. Call this energy what you will – God, your spirit, the universe, Brahman, source energy, Allah, Yahweh, the quantum field, etc. – the real "you" is non-physical, and that is becoming more difficult to deny.

Tool #3, meditation, allows you to meet the real "you," the non-physical you, and learn from your own wisdom. This tool helps you achieve your ideal weight because being in contact with the real you, your non-physical energy, helps you feel calmer, more secure, more confident, more serene, more at peace, and happier. And feeling that way is like rocket fuel for all the other tools and rules of losing your unwanted weight and keeping it off.

The good news is that all the benefits of meditation are simple to achieve – they only take willingness and practice. And practicing meditation requires, at most, 15 minutes a day.

Most of what I know about meditation is an amalgamation of what I've learned from Dr. Dyer and Dr. Chopra. There are many methods of meditation and many philosophies about it. Feel free to do whatever makes you most comfortable, even if your practice differs from mine. Ultimately, the most important thing about meditation is to still your mind, and however you find yourself best able to do that is wonderful.

Stilling your mind means choosing not to listen to the incessant chatter that your brain throws at you all day long. It has been said that your non-physical energy can be found in the empty space between your thoughts. Meditation can be seen simply as an effective effort to widen the space between your thoughts. When you find the space between your thoughts, you'll find your true self – your non-physical "you" – and it is in perfect alignment with all your dreams.

And here's a big reveal:

The real, non-physical "you" has no unwanted weight and is actually excited about the physical "you" experiencing your ideal weight!

The way I meditate is very simple. I find a quiet spot and sit cross-legged, with my hands resting, upturned, on my knees and my thumbs and middle fingers touching. I close my eyes and imagine I'm sitting alone in a movie theater (there's that movie metaphor again). On the movie screen are the two words "I" and "Love." Then, in my mind's eye, I focus upon the empty space between the "I" and the "Love," all the while imagining good feelings shooting up my spine and escaping into the universe. When other thoughts arise, I don't freak out or get upset; I simply imagine a mild breeze is blowing through my mind and gently whisking away my thoughts without any trouble.

Another method you might enjoy is to sit in the same comfortable style I just described and then imagine you're taking the top of your skull off, reaching into your cranium, and gently removing your brain. In your imagination, gently set your brain down beside you (I literally make the movements with my hands when I'm doing this) and lovingly tell your brain, "I'm not going to need you for the next fifteen minutes or so, my friend." Then sit quietly as a person with no brain and, therefore, no thoughts.

I do this for 15 minutes each day, preferably in the morning before I start into my daily routines and responsibilities. I want you to do it for 15 minutes each day, too. When you meditate, do so with no agendas or planned outcomes. Your goal is simply to spend as much of the 15 minutes as possible without thought, which is how you commune with your non-physical "you."

You'll find that, when you meditate, you're listening to the wisdom of the real "you," and that wisdom will often come in the form of feelings rather than words. Another wonderful benefit from your meditation practice is that the better you get at listening and communing with the real "you," the better you'll be able to listen to your gut and your instincts when it comes to eating and moving. You'll fool yourself into doing things that make you feel badly much less often because you're more in tune with your true nature and how you really feel. If you're like me, you're going to find yourself falling in love with your non-physical energy – which really means you'll be falling in love with yourself!

Tool #4: Still Your Mind as Often as Possible

"The activities we observe in the outer world are but typical of that which is taking place in man's inner world of thought and feeling."

Charles Patterson
Author

As you practice meditation each day and commune with your non-physical energy, you will find yourself wanting to spend more and more time in between your thoughts because of all the freedom you find there. The energy of you, found in the empty space between your thoughts, is infinite, unbounded, and loving. It not only feels good spending time there, but being in touch with it also acts as a catalyst for making your dreams become real.

In your case, of course, you wish to lose your unwanted weight and keep it off. This is a desire you've had for many years, and it has constantly eluded you because you spent most of your energy focused upon your actions rather than making sure you feel good about your actions before you do them. But trust me, the energy of the universe has heard your desire to lose your unwanted weight. In fact, the universe has your ideal body just waiting for you to allow it to happen by becoming friends with eating and moving.

The good news is that becoming friends with eating and moving is exactly what you're doing right now, by following the three simple rules about those activities. And the even better news is that, even before it has become second nature for you to tell good stories about eating and moving, there is a way to experience all the benefits of a completely positive, uplifting state of being.

In the absence of your telling nothing but good stories about all the eating and moving you do, you can do something just as powerful: tell *no* stories at all. Stilling your mind is just that: telling no stories. And when you still your mind, you have effectively turned off your brain and are making no judgments at all, which allows the universe to deliver to you all it has waiting for you in storage.

Stilling your mind is a form of waking, interactive meditation. The way you still your mind can be very simple. Just keep your attention on your environment while you imagine a cool breeze blowing the thoughts right out of your head. You don't have to withdraw from your normal, daily activity to do this.

An additional way to still your mind works very well when driving. After all, you probably drive quite a bit each day so this is a great opportunity for you to practice this tool. As I described in the previous tool, "Meditate for 15 Minutes Each Day", imagine you're taking the top of your skull off, reaching into your cranium, and gently removing your brain. In your imagination, gently set your brain down beside you (I literally make the movements with my hands when I'm doing this) and lovingly tell your brain, "I'm not going to need you for the next fifteen minutes or so, my friend." Then drive without thought or judgment (while still paying attention to traffic, road signs, and directions).

You can still your mind anytime during your day for as long or as brief a time as you can get away with. And every time you still your mind, you will be in direct communion with your non-physical energy – the real "you" who is waiting to present you with your ideal body as soon as you'll allow it to happen.

I like to think of it this way. Your blocked, unrealized desires (like your ideal weight) are waiting for you in a giant lake of unrealized potential (the quantum field). The dam creating this lake is your resistance, your brain constantly telling bad stories that focus on "Where is it? It isn't here!" That dam is the only thing standing between you and your ideal weight — and any other desires you have yet to see come to fruition.

Each time you still your mind, you open a spigot that allows your blocked desires to begin flowing into your life experience. By stilling your mind, you neutralize all the negativity and resistance that is blocking your desires. How much flows and how long it flows out of that giant lake of blocked desires depends on how long and how often you still your mind each day.

In addition, you'll love the clarity and serenity you gain from stilling your mind. Shutting off your brain's constant clatter, if only for a few moments, can be like taking a long nap. It is incredibly refreshing and invigorating. And the more time you spend bonding with your true, non-physical self, the more confidence you'll feel in the new you taking shape.

Tool #5: Feel Gratitude as Often as Possible

"The greatest discovery of my generation is that human beings can alter their lives by altering their attitudes of mind."

William James
Psychologist

Of all the feelings in the world, there may be nothing more powerful than gratitude. If it were possible to feel gratitude at all times, I have no doubt that you would be a superhuman who made your desires manifest almost instantly. If you have any doubts about this, practice feeling gratitude as often as possible for a while and you'll soon see for yourself.

With this tool, you are now introduced to the most powerful tool imaginable for crafting good-feeling stories that serve you rather than hinder and block you.

Gratitude makes your stories feel amazingly good. And the good news is, you can feel grateful for anything and for any reason. To start, begin by looking at things you've become accustomed to taking for granted. Certainly your ability to breath, walk, talk, imagine, love, eat, and dream are just a few things that you can choose to feel grateful for right now. After all, you aren't *guaranteed* that you'll continue to have any of those gifts you are currently enjoying.

It's impossible to feel gratitude without feeling good.

When you have had a taste of gratitude for the "little things" you once habitually took for granted, move on to gratitude for the "small" victories. Eating one doughnut instead of three before you realize you don't feel good about it is something to be grateful for. Sure, you can beat yourself up for eating the one doughnut, but doesn't finding gratitude in your *growth* feel better? And isn't beating yourself up a cardinal "no-no" for all your eating and moving rules anyway?

Going outside today and walking around your block when you haven't done so in years is cause for gratitude, too. Who cares if you didn't do it at a record pace? Pat your back and say, "Way to go, me!" Feel grateful for the movement you did rather than feeling bad for having walked "only a block."

As you begin feeling grateful for the "little things" you once called "not enough," you'll really be on the track to greatness. For example, I may not run as much as a really dedicated athlete, but I am grateful for my ability and opportunities to go on a two- or three-mile jog! Nobody (except me) can tell me that's not enough movement! And, because I'm choosing to be grateful for all my movement today, I know I'm doing enough.

Once you've gotten practice feeling grateful for the things you once took for granted and for the "little" things that once felt like they weren't enough, you'll be ready for the major leagues of gratitude. Here, you'll start telling yourself the best stories you can ever imagine. Gratitude will become almost your secret super-power! You can now begin to completely make your own rules about being grateful.

For example, spiritualists and physicists alike both teach us that two opposite experiences, such as "giving" and "receiving," are really *the same exact experience* – they are just being viewed from two different perspectives.

This example shows you that you are free to make your own rules. You can actually choose to be grateful for anything you experience (yes, even the "unwanted" things) if you decide to see it as merely the opposite perspective of something you desire more. Another example is finding gratitude in experiences you would normally label bad because you choose to see them as necessary contrasting experiences that are showing you what you <u>don't want</u>, motivating you to make the changes necessary to get what you <u>do want</u>.

By making your own rules for gratitude, you can begin to actually feel grateful for your unwanted weight. Sound crazy? Who made the rules that you have to feel *bad* about your unwanted weight and that you can't feel grateful for it? Later, I'll reveal why I'm so grateful for any unwanted weight I've had. I'll suggest that, if you so choose, you can find reasons to feel grateful for your unwanted weight – perhaps because it's given you motivation and a reason to learn and grow in unexpected ways.

I extend my right to feel grateful for anything I choose to all areas of my life. If you're like me, you'll learn that no one will punish you, scold you, or put you in time-out for feeling grateful about anything. In fact, if you're like me, you'll be infused with energy and a connection to the real, non-physical you when you remember to be grateful. You, too, may find that gratitude is addictive because of the way feeling good about yourself brings wonderful results into your life.

I promise you that when you get to the point where you are looking for ways to feel grateful for most things you experience (and you will, with practice) you will be well on your way to never having to experience any unwanted weight again.

Tool #6: Create and Celebrate Success

"A person is what he or she thinks about all day long."

Ralph Waldo Emerson
Author

The sixth tool, Create and Celebrate Success, picks up where practicing gratitude left off. A commitment to practicing gratitude leads to creating successes. And practicing gratitude also leads to celebrating your successes. Creating and celebrating your success, in turn, presents more and more opportunities for gratitude. And that's a wonderful circle to be caught up in!

One of my Father's favorite Smile Strategies is "Celebrate Everything." That's because celebrating everything gives you the greatest opportunity to feel grateful and appreciative. With this tool, I am asking you to take celebrating yourself and your accomplishments to uncharted territory. Similar to what I asked you to do with gratitude, I want you to *create* things to celebrate – simply because you can! Because celebrating will fill you with positive energy and open yourself up to receive even more from your reservoir of blocked desires.

I want you to celebrate things you would normally have barely acknowledged, such as eating a bowl of fresh fruit for breakfast rather than some food you would normally feel bad about eating, or someone complimenting you on how you look. Pump up the volume for such events and pat yourself on the back till you're sore! In fact, I recommend that you *literally* pat yourself on the back. As you start doing this more and more, you'll start to feel like your own biggest fan and you'll find that's an incredible motivation to keep moving forward.

Also begin to look for celebrations you would have normally overlooked but that recognize a change in the stories you're telling and a change in your behavior. Celebrate things like *not* looking at yourself in the mirror, *not* weighing yourself, saying something nice about yourself when you <u>do</u> see your reflection, referring to yourself kindly. Celebrate the times you think, "I have unwanted weight" instead of "I am fat." Celebrate feeling a little excitement about your opportunities for movement. Celebrate *anytime* you tell a better feeling story!

Think about how you teach a child to ride a bike. You wouldn't put her on a bike and say, "Go to it" while you watched from the porch, would you? And you certainly wouldn't chastise her when she messed up and fell over. You'd encourage and celebrate every little bit of progress she made, starting with her being able to sit on the bike seat, to her pedaling for a few feet (even with your steady hand on her back). Celebrating a child's successes helps her gain confidence and build a skill that you know she'll eventually master. But there's only one way to get there: by practicing. By making mistakes and experiencing one little success after another until, finally, she reaches her goal!

You know that the best way to teach a child is not to chastise her for making a mistake. So why not give yourself that same nurturing care and encouragement? Anticipate your desire to celebrate success on your journey to your ideal weight. Plan achievable goals and also plan to celebrate those achievements. As you walk your block for the first time, celebrate by meeting friends for coffee later that day. As you eat a salad for lunch instead of a burger and fries, celebrate by seeing a funny movie that evening.

And lose the requirement that others join in with you. Who cares if no one else wants to celebrate with you or even if people pooh-pooh your celebrating as frivolous? Feel sorry for them and continue! And, if you need to, simply keep your celebrations private.

Take celebrating seriously and you'll see seriously good results from it. More gratitude. More energy. Greater and faster loss of unwanted weight. In fact, a great way to use this tool is to cultivate a group of friends to whom you can openly and wantonly "brag" about yourself without having to apologize or throw in statements of unnecessary humility. Get some friends who'll let you toot your own horn as loudly and proudly as you can while understanding that you're doing it because it's good to celebrate yourself.

Chapter Eighteen - The End? No Way! This is Just the Beginning!

"When you change the way you look at things, the things you look at change."

Max Planck

Physicist

Nobel Prize Winner

It took me 15 years to achieve my ideal body. You'll arrive much sooner, because you won't have to make all the mistakes I did. And not only will you achieve your ideal weight and be able to maintain it, in doing so you will enter the prime of your life! As a good friend of mine who lost over 100 pounds using these principles likes to say, "If, when I started this lifestyle, I'd written down everything I *thought* I'd get out of it, I'd have severely shortchanged myself!"

Here's a good example of how changing my paradigms and my stories about eating worked for me. I used to talk and obsess about whether food was bad for me. I counted calories, carbohydrates, and fat grams. Then I would deprive myself of all the good-tasting food that I craved because it was bad for me to eat. Consequently, I would force myself to eat the bad-tasting food I didn't want because I thought it was good for me to eat it. Bear in mind that I was the sole source of, and bore full responsibility for, my stories of what foods were good and what foods were bad. Certainly, I based my stories on diet and nutrition literature, but it was I who made the choice to adopt and believe those stories.

Now you might say, "But that literature was written by licensed, credentialed experts who knew their stuff about food and health. Doesn't that mean I *should* have listened to them and believed them?" And I will counter by reminding you that our universe does not work on action but on energy. So the real question is *not* whether I should have believed the stories of the experts but whether I felt good about the stories I was telling myself based on that literature. And my answer to that question was a resounding no. The stories I told myself after listening to the food experts did not feel good.

So, under these circumstances, I was faced with two choices: Either I stopped eating any foods about which I couldn't tell any good-feeling stories or I learned to tell better feeling stories about foods I wished to continue eating. Since I believed the experts were correct about fresh vegetables and fruit being good for my body and fat and excess calories being bad for my body, I chose to begin telling myself better feeling stories about fresh vegetables and fruit!

By this point, I was eating fresh fruit in the morning instead of doughnuts or pancakes (some of my old favorites), but I just didn't naturally feel good about eating fresh fruit. It did not feel realistic to tell myself a story like "I love eating fresh fruits and I never want to go back to eating doughnuts and pancakes in the morning! I am so glad I have found this wonderful new way to eat in the morning!" But I *was* able to tell myself a story like "*Just for today*, I am willing to eat fresh fruit this morning. I give myself permission to decide again tomorrow whether I want to continue, but I can do this for <u>one day</u>." I told myself that story each morning for weeks and I *did* begin to slowly feel better about eating fresh fruit.

"Everything is possible for him who believes."

Mark 9:23

The Bible

But I didn't stop there. After a week or so, I began to add to my story: "And I can also believe that it's possible for me to start <u>enjoying</u> the consumption of fresh fruit just as much as I enjoy the consumption of doughnuts and pancakes. I don't enjoy fruit as much right now, but I'm willing to believe that I can eventually." At that point, that better-feeling story felt realistic, and I soon felt *even better* about eating all that fresh fruit.

As my good feelings about eating fresh fruit grew, it started to feel realistic to add still more good-feeling stories, such as "I am pretty confident that I can find fruits that I enjoy during each season and, perhaps, even come to anticipate the arrival of them as their season approaches." That story felt great, and by this time, after months of eating fresh fruit, it felt completely believable. And, for the first time in my life, I was actually excited about eating fresh fruit.

As my feelings improved and I was no longer spending anywhere near the energy telling myself bad-feeling stories about missing the old foods, I started to experience different results with my body. My beliefs and, thus, my expectations, were changing and the universe was responding in small but noticeable ways. For example, I noticed I had more physical energy since starting to eat fresh fruit in the morning. In addition, I began to see that some of my unwanted weight was leaving. I also felt proud of myself for nourishing my body so lovingly.

Momentum was building!

Within six months, I was telling myself stories like "I love eating fresh fruits and I *never* want to go back to eating doughnuts and pancakes in the morning! I am so glad I have found this wonderful new way to eat in the mornings!" And I <u>knew</u> these stories were true to the core of my soul! They had become my reality; I had successfully changed my beliefs! And I had done it one story at a time – not trying to jump up to the best feeling stories at first, but working my way up by telling myself the best feeling stories *that felt believable* to me every step of the way.

I did the same thing with fresh vegetables, organic foods, healthier options when eating out, and eating less fat, salt, and grease. I now honestly do not even *like* to eat anything but fresh fruit in the mornings. I love fresh vegetables (steamed and without any butter on them) and I do not like fast food anymore at all. These good feelings about such healthy fare reflect my new beliefs. They serve me and uplift me and they feel fantastic! I almost never feel deprived anymore, nor do I have to *force* myself to stick to any certain diet, because I have learned to feel great about what I eat!

And, yes, I am able to eat ice cream and doughnuts today. I have learned how to eat those foods in moderation and feel good about doing it.

And I did it by telling myself the best possible stories about my eating, starting with how I really felt and slowly improving those stories over time to the point where I now have some phenomenal beliefs about eating that really serve me and my body beautifully. My beliefs have allowed me to take off all my unwanted weight. Gone! And I have kept it off, with ease, for about 14 years now.

I had very similar experiences with the movement aspect of this plan.

I have run since I was 14, competitively in school and recreationally as an adult. But usually, while running, I told myself stories such as "This is hard" or "I can't wait to get this over with" or "Oh crud, here comes another hill." I clearly remember that, most of the time, I had to *make* myself go out and run, because I believed running <u>was</u> difficult and I <u>didn't</u> enjoy it! Those were the stories I told myself repeatedly and, because of that, those were my beliefs.

Consequently, my desired manifestations from jogging were frustratingly elusive. I was never really the lean, strong athlete I wanted to be. It felt like I was always fighting against something when I ran and that my desired results were always just out of my reach.

For the last six years, I have chosen to tell the best story possible while I jog. I started saying things to myself (telling stories) like "This is great" and "Thank you for this opportunity to move my body" and "Oh darn. Only two more hills after this one; I love hills!"

And, over time, I've created new beliefs about jogging just the same way I did about eating – one story at a time. You know how I can tell? Because, unlike my previous experiences as a younger man, I now get excited when I think about going on a run! Because jogging is <u>fun</u> and it <u>is</u> a wonderful gift to move my body. Those are my beliefs now!

The quantum field always gives you what

you believe and expect. Whatever you believe, the quantum field always gives it to you exactly as you expect it. It can be frustrating to realize, however, that what you expect and what you desire can be two different things.

"In fact, it is often stated that all of the theories proposed in this century, the silliest is quantum theory. Some say that only thing that quantum theory has going for it, in fact, is that it is unquestionably correct."

Michio Kaku
Physicist

My new beliefs (and expectations) about eating and moving have almost *nothing* to do with any actions. As quantum physics teaches us, it's not about the action - its about the energy. To summarize:

We hold beliefs.

Our beliefs create our expectations.

The quantum field delivers exactly what we expect (which, as you know, is not always in alignment with what we desire).

Our feelings tell us whether our beliefs are in alignment with our desires. If we feel good, we are in alignment; if we feel bad, we aren't.

Your feelings are like your thermometer – telling you how much your beliefs and your desires are in (or out) of alignment. Good feelings let you know that your beliefs and desires are aligned, while bad feelings let you know that your beliefs and desires are not aligned. And how intense the good or bad feeling is indicates how closely aligned (or how greatly separated) your beliefs and desires are.

The solution to being out of alignment with your beliefs is to change what you know. You do this by consistently deciding to always tell yourself the best story you can possibly believe.

Practice telling the best story possible about all the people, places, things, and circumstances you encounter and, over time, you will find that your feelings will change about lots of things. Things about your body that used to automatically signal you to feel like a loser, unlucky, or down in the dumps won't make you feel so bad. You'll be training yourself to see more and more clearly the gifts and blessings inherent in everything. And as your feelings change about eating and moving (from your practice of telling the best story possible), your beliefs, too, will change!

As your beliefs become more closely aligned with your desires, you will feel optimism, find gratitude, and you will see the gifts in almost all your life's circumstances. And you will experience much more of what you want from life, including a new and beautiful body. That is because, as your beliefs change, the universe will change with them. As you feel better about yourself, you will manifest things more and more closely aligned with your desires. Even relationships, peace, serenity, career opportunities, health, and self-acceptance can be found, as the joys of the universe automatically manifest in response to your new beliefs.

This process, as described in this chapter, is your prescription for using the amazing science of quantum physics in your life, right now, to change yourself and your world. By following this process you are, literally, plugged in to the way the universe really functions. Through the two new paradigms (energy-based and holism), you will not and, in fact, cannot fail because quantum physics is so wonderfully and incredibly accurate and precise. You are being that superhuman you fantasized about in the "What if…" Chapter!

"Imagination is everything. It is the preview of life's coming attractions"

Albert Einstein
Physicist
Nobel Prize Winner

And, if you're like me, you will discover that the quantum field has always been infinite, abundant, and ready to deliver all those wonderful things to you. Even when you felt your worst about yourself, those things were still available to you because they are your birthright! The stream of good will didn't <u>increase</u> through your practice of telling better stories (it couldn't *get* any larger!); only the *size* of the bucket you dip into the stream of good will increased!

You see, <u>you</u> are the bucket that gets dipped into the universe's stream of good will. And the size of your bucket is dictated by how much self-worth you feel; the greater your self-worth, the bigger the bucket you dip into the stream! Now that your self-worth is on the rise, you're going to be shouting with joy, "Fill 'er up, universe!"

And you're going to love what you find, ideal body and all.

About the Author

Author Greg Kuhn is a professional educator and a futurist, specializing in framing new paradigms for 21st Century living. Since 1995, he has written primarily with his father, Dr. Clifford Kuhn, M.D., about health, wellness, and productivity.

Greg Kuhn lives in Louisville, KY with a wonderful wife and four fantastic sons (one by marriage) whom he, literally, couldn't have published this book without; you can read more at http://whyquantumphysicists.wordpress.com/ and http://www.squidoo.com/why-quantum-physicists-dont-get-fat.

Future books in Greg's "Why Quantum Physicists..." series will cover:

- Teaching
- School success
- Financial abundance
- Romantic relationships
- Parenting

Greg gives talks and presentations for these topics, tailored for both adult and youth audiences; if you'd like to inquire about his availability simply email him at Laughdrjr@insightbb.com and/or contact him through the sites previously listed. Feel free, also, to contact Greg and suggest additional topics for his "Why Quantum Physicists…" series.

33600185R00110

Made in the USA
Lexington, KY
01 July 2014